ADVOCATING FOR OTHERS:
A POCKET RESOURCE FOR PEER
SPECIALISTS AND COUNSELORS

ADVOCATING FOR OTHERS: A POCKET RESOURCE FOR PEER SPECIALISTS AND COUNSELORS

Charles Drebing, PhD

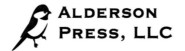

ALDERSON PRESS, LLC

Alderson Press, LLC
15 Church Place
Holliston, MA 01746

Library of Congress Cataloging in Publication Data
Drebing, Charles, 1959–
Advocating for Others: A Pocket Resource for Peer Specialists
and Counselors
/ by Charles E. Drebing
ISBN 978-1-329-80309-1

To all of the advocates who have worked to change the healthcare and social service systems for adults and children who suffer with mental illness. Their persistent hope results in better lives for many people and better places to work for many providers.

CONTENTS

PREFACE

One of my first tasks as a manager for a large mental health organization was to attend a monthly consumer council meeting within our PTSD program. "You will need to wear protective armor" a friend told me. "They are experienced consumers and they are TOUGH!!!" I felt warned and a little anxious as I joined this group of Veterans who had been serving as advocates for the hundreds of others receiving services in this program.

The warning was accurate -- they were tough advocates. They knew about real problems and they wanted those problems addressed. Initially I found myself getting anxious before each meeting, as I knew that they were going to raise concerns, some of which I had heard about in the past, some of which would be new. What made me more anxious is that I knew that they would ask for updates about the prior concerns that they had raised. Some problems I had been able to resolve, and that always felt satisfying to report. Often, the problems were not easily solved, and so I had to report on my partial success and my continuing efforts.

At times, they would ask that front-line staff be included in the discussion, as they knew that the frontline staff played a key role in how care was provided, and knew a great deal about the problems that needed to change. When we invited frontline staff, I often felt that another key set of advocates had been included. Frontline staff often knows much more about what is really happening than managers. They see the problems and the successes. They deal with the underlying causes every day. They are also intensely committed to solving the problems they face. I grew to value them as natural advocates and partners.

Over the first three years working together, despite my discomfort -- possibly because of it -- we got a lot accomplished. We changed the way those we serve heard about services, how they participated in treatment decisions, and how programs worked with clients moving between services. We improved communication. We also worked on things that I had not anticipated, like parking, signage, and furniture. I had to learn about a wide range of things that no clinical training prepared me for. My experience with that consumer council taught me some key lessons:

- Consumers/clients and their advocates (Peers and frontline staff) have a lot of feelings about the services provided, some of which clinicians and managers can anticipate, but some of which they have no idea about.

- What advocates think will improve care is often very different from what professional clinicians think will improve care. Consumers and their advocates often identify basic elements of care (how engaged clinicians are, how respectful staff are, how collaborative/flexible they are) and practical issues (parking, waiting, communication) related to their experience, while clinicians tend to focus on the latest models of care - the newest medications, therapies or technology.

- Consumers, and particularly those who serve as advocates, know a great deal about the practical operations of a clinical program. They talk to each other, and so collect a great deal of information about the experience of many people. They often know about problems that are not obvious to staff and particularly not to managers.

- Advocates tend to be very effective at disseminating information. The same channels they use to collect information, work to spread information to the broader group of consumers. Advocates tend to be opinion-leaders in any client group, and so not only do they disseminate information, but they influence the attitude that clients have toward the organization.

- The pressure that advocates bring to the table is helpful - it results in improvements that are important and that often won't happen without them. That pressure is not always comfortable, and can generate more work for managers and for programs, but in the end produces meaningful improvement.

- Over time, advocates become a key strategic partner to any clinician and manager. Regular interactions between staff and experienced advocates will produce real results in terms of improvements in care and in the experience of the client.

- Not all advocates have the same skills, and so not all are equally helpful. This is no surprise, as they usually have limited training if any, in how to serve as an advocate.

My recognition of the value of advocates and the lack of formal training available for advocates is the motivation for this book. After I realized how valuable advocates were to me as a manager, I looked for ways to support their development of the skills that make them most effective.

My hope is that those of you who serve as advocates, whether you are a Peer Support Specialist, a member of a consumer council or a frontline clinical staff member, will recognize the importance of the advocacy work that naturally comes to you, and recognize that you are needed by the organization you serve. The organizations may not always communicate that to you, but know that you are their partner and a key part of the solution to their desire to be effective. Also know that advocacy, like any complex role, involves a variety of skills that need to be developed. Some of you will have natural skills and will excel at aspects of advocacy from the start. Most will have to work to develop those skills. Everyone will get better by thinking about how they do this work (thus this book) and by gaining more and more experience as advocates.

ACKNOWLEDGMENTS

Special thanks to Tom Raposa, Tracy Claudio and the PTSD
Consumer Council for modeling each day what effective
advocacy looks like. Additional thanks to Laurel Holland whose
creative support was of great help and to Heather Rodino for her
exceptional input and editorial assistance.

HOW TO USE THIS BOOK

This book is specifically designed for Peer Specialists and frontline counselors who serve as advocates as part of their work with adults receiving mental health and/or substance-use services. Written to serve as an easy-to-access pocket resource, it provides basic information you need to know in order to be an effective advocate. Keep it at hand and reference it as you work.

Advocacy within healthcare and social service settings can take many shapes. Some efforts involve no more than a phone call, while others require a team to work for years to achieve a large-scale goal. In this book, you'll find general strategies relevant to the full range of situations you may encounter. You'll also find guidance on some advanced advocacy skills that you might want to develop. You will need to adopt—and adapt—these strategies for the advocacy work that you typically do.

This book is also designed to supply specific information that advocates may need to help them find partnering organizations quickly, and to share that information with the people they advocate for. Some of these details will need to be customized for the setting in which you work and your area of the country. For this reason, you'll be asked to fill in key phone numbers, contacts, referral sources, and information so that it will be easily available to you while you are working (see chapter 17).

Advocating for Others is a basic resource tool, and is not meant to replace more complete resources or education on advocacy. If you will be working as an advocate, you may want to look for larger resources and educational opportunities. Nor is this book a substitute for learning the guidelines and policies of the organization you work for. It does, however, include additional links and contacts that can help you continue your growth in this important role.

A Note on Critical Situations That Advocates May Uncover.
Advocates are asked to help people who are often facing
significant challenges, including some situations which may
include a serious crisis. It is also not uncommon for advocates to
uncover other very serious problems as they are talking with the
people they are serving. When this happens, it is critical that
advocates are able to respond effectively to these situations,
whether it is a person at risk for hurting themselves or others, or
someone who is aware of someone in immediate danger.
Appendix A has been included as a quick guide to help you
respond to these types of critical situations.

CHAPTER 1

WHAT IS ADVOCACY?

To advocate is to recommend, support, plead for, argue for, or bring pressure to bear in support of a cause or proposal. Advocates can be a wide range of people who push for something that they want to happen, using a wide range of strategies. Advocacy may refer to small actions like making a simple request for someone else (e.g. Asking if a standard procedure can be changed to better serve a client) or a large and extended action (e.g. Working with a team of advocates to get the state mental health budget increased). Improvements in any system are not typically made unless someone recognizes the need and pushes for them. When someone pushes for the welfare of others, that person is acting as an advocate.

Peer Support Specialists, often referred to as "Peers," are people who have personal experience with recovery from a mental health and/or substance-use problem, and are willing to talk about that experience in order to help others. Patients and clients engaged in treatment naturally look to Peers to help address challenges they face in obtaining care, so these individuals are well positioned to serve as advocates.

I use the term "counselors" to refer to any clinical professionals, many of whom often serve as frontline staff, who provide a range of services in mental health and social service settings. They may have varied educational backgrounds, but what they share is a common goal of helping adults use mental health and/or social services as a way of reaching recovery. From their perspective, they often see the challenges their clients face, including those that may be created by the system of care.

I use the term "stakeholder" to refer to any person or group that has an investment or interest in the success of the services being provided. The most obvious stakeholders are the clients, their families and friends, and the clinical and administrative staff from the organization providing the services. Less obvious are those stakeholders who also serve the clients (e.g. other oranizations or programs that serve the same group) and stakeholders who have a broader "stake" in the effectiveness of the service (e.g. the community, taxpayers and other funding sources, advocacy and professional organizations).

Because of their experience, Peer Specialists and counselors often have the best perspective of all groups of stakeholders, for identifying problems that clients may face in getting the care they need, and the potential solutions to those problems. They also often have ongoing relationships with other staff and administrators of healthcare and social service organizations. The combination of these relationships, their clinical experience, and the respect Peers and frontline staff have earned from other stakeholders puts them in an ideal position for advocating for change. Unfortunately, most Peer Specialists and counselors have not been formally trained to be advocates, may not recognize situations when advocacy is needed, and may not have the skills to advocate successfully when they do.

ADVOCATING VS. EMPOWERING CLIENTS

In most situations in which clients want or need providers to change some practice or resource, the appropriate first step is to help those clients pursue that change themselves. The clients may need guidance and encouragement, but it is in their interest to be the one's requesting a change, and working with the provider or agency to achieve that change. By empowering our clients to be their own change agents, we help further their recovery, while encouraging the natural constructive collaboration between clients and providers.

Peer Specialists and counselors get involved as advocates when clients are unable to ask for the change, or when the need for change is broader or more complex than is reflected by the needs of just one client.

COMMON WAYS THAT PEER SPECIALISTS AND COUNSELORS ADVOCATE

1. <u>Advocating for Individuals Receiving Services from a Specific Healthcare or Social Service Provider.</u> Clinicians and social service providers usually have to work collaboratively with their clients for a positive outcome to occur. And so it is particularly important when situations arise in which providers and clients disagree and/or have difficulty working together. When clients or providers are not good at collaborating, disagreements are even more likely.
When a disagreement arises, a number of factors can make it particularly difficult for some providers to recognize the needs of clients. Providers are often trained to take on the role of "expert," offering opinions based on extensive training. They also have more experience with the range of clinical situations than their clients. Thus, by the nature of their role and their broader experience, they have more explicit power and may

feel more confident in their own opinion. This can cause
them to miss the important truth that the client is at the
center of the care, and they typically have the best perspective
on what the goal and the experience of treatment are. When
communication and understanding break down, then the
shared efforts of both clients and providers suffer. Advocates
can help level the playing field, making it easier for clients to
be heard and to be active in managing their own care.

2. Advocating for an Individual or Group of People with a
   Healthcare or Social Service Program or Organization.
   Sometimes it is not the provider, but the program or
   organization that needs to change. Without advocates, clients
   often feel that they don't know how to request changes and
   have little chance of being heard.   Peer advocates can be
   effective voices, asking for review and revision of program
   and organizational practices in order to improve the care
   clients receive.

3. Serving on or Leading a Consumer Council Within a
   Healthcare or Social Service Program or Organization.
   Consumer councils are common structures in healthcare and
   social service organizations. They are designed to gather data
   about consumer needs and desires and to push for
   improvement in services. Peer advocates in particular, are
   ideal members of these councils, as they know the clients'
   perspective and experiences, and have experience in helping
   organizations change.   Clinical staff are often valuable as
   consumer council liaisons, listening to the concerns raised by
   council members, and providing background information so
   that the council understands the background to their concern.

4. Serving as a Member of an Advocacy Organization. A growing
   number of organizations that have advocacy as their primary
   mission are staffed by Peer Specialists. These organizations

engage in a wide range of advocacy activities and are becoming a valuable voice in changing large and small aspects of the healthcare and social service system.

5. <u>Lobbying Key Organizational or Political Leaders.</u>
Organizational and political leaders are often most influenced by personal stories about how problems and changes impact the lives of real people. Peer Specialists and clinical professionals are very well suited to talk about personal stories—those of their clients and themselves—and so have a great deal to offer to lobbying efforts.

Your advocacy work may include many of these roles or just one. Fortunately, the skills required to be successful in each role tend to be the same, though they will need some adaptation. Experience across advocacy roles and settings will help speed your skill development, so look for those opportunities. Despite the variations in advocacy across these roles, there are some basic boundaries on what advocates do and don't do. Consider the following basic guidelines.

Advocates Do	Advocates Don't
Seek to help people in recovery by finding ways to encourage change in practices and decisions that impact the recovery of those they serve.	Passively accept barriers to recovery resulting from the actions (or lack of action) of providers, without trying to change them.
Encourage clients to advocate for themselves, and get involved only when it is clear that those clients need additional assistance or the issue is larger than a single client or group of clients.	Undermine clients' sense of empowerment by stepping in when they could take action themselves to solve their own problems.

Advocates Do	Advocates Don't
Believe and express hope that situations, individuals, and organizations can improve.	Believe or express hopelessness in the face of barriers to recovery.
Choose a strategy for advocating that matches the goal and the people or organizations they are working with.	Advocate without thinking through which strategy will be most effective for meeting the goals of those they are serving.
Build positive relationships over time with both clients and the organizations, programs and people they are advocating to.	Ignore the long-term impact of what they are doing, just focusing on the short-term goal of "winning" the issue in front of them.
Act in a way that is trustworthy and ethical.	Act in ways that indicate they are—or appear to be— untrustworthy, dishonest, or unethical. Hold or express higher expectations for others than they do for themselves.
Stay in communication and follow-up with the person or group they are advocating for.	Lose track of the person or group they are serving by failing to communicate or follow-up.

CHAPTER 2

THE ADVOCATE'S STANCE

When you are serving as an advocate, you have a different role than you would usually as a Peer Specialist or a clinician. Part of being a good advocate is developing a feel for that role—the way to think, talk, and act like an advocate. The following guidelines will help you to be clear about how you should approach your work.

1. <u>Maintain a Clear Focus on Helping Someone or Some Group in Recovery.</u> Advocacy is primarily a means of pushing for change. Many other opportunities and agendas arise while advocating for someone, but the effective advocate maintains a keen focus on the priority of the person or group being served. Effective advocates do not get distracted or diverted from their goal.

2. <u>Recognize That Change Often Requires Pressure.</u> Desired changes rarely happen by chance—it is people who change things, often in response to pressures and incentives. The type of pressure that advocates exert can take many forms. Each form represents a tool that an effective advocate chooses to use to address a specific situation. At its foundation, advocacy

is the process of bringing different types of pressure to bear in an effort to persuade others to change something.

3. <u>Recognize the Power of Advocacy.</u> Successful advocates do not take the power of their role lightly and are careful not to misuse it. Whenever pressure is being exerted, there is usually a cost. This might take the shape of resistance or resentment among some of those being pushed, or a change in the relationship between the client and the target of the advocacy. Effective advocates recognize the cost and include it in their decisions about how to advocate.

4. <u>Work from a Foundation of Recovery Values.</u> Advocates gain their legitimacy because they are serving the goal of recovery. Working in a way that contradicts or ignores recovery values often leads to failure over time, as other stakeholders lose confidence that the advocate is working for something they can buy into.

- <u>Hope.</u> Advocates maintain hope both that their client(s) can get better *and* that the target of their advocacy can improve. Advocates also maintain hope that their advocacy target wants to act in the client's best interest and that part of the process is to help others see how change is in everyone's interest.

- <u>Honesty.</u> The long-term effectiveness of any advocate depends heavily on the trust built among both the people the individual advocates for and with. While short-term gains can be made by less-than-honest strategies, the loss of trust is rarely worth it.

- <u>Responsibility.</u> Effective advocates recognize that everyone in the situation has responsibilities: those they are advocating for, those they are advocating with, and they - the advocates. Taking a visibly responsible stance and talking about everyone's responsibilities will encourage all to live up to their duties.

- Respect. Similarly, everyone in the advocacy situation deserves respect. Effective advocates show respect and expect respect for their clients, those they advocate to, and themselves. They are attentive to how they and others communicate respect and the implications of these messages.

- Realism. Effective advocates maintain a keen focus on the real-life issues that their clients are facing and the real benefits they are seeking. By avoiding getting into entrenched symbolic battles, the advocate ensures that practical benefits for the client will the primary result.

- Patience and Persistence. Change often takes time. Many of the most important changes are achieved by long-term pressure, and so the persistent advocate is often the one who achieves the most significant changes for clients.

5. Recognize the Range of Skills Needed: Work Toward Developing Those Skills and Use Them Strategically. Like any skilled craftsman, the effective advocate has a variety of skills and strategies and uses them when the proper situation arises. The advocate builds those skills through education and training, and by watching oneself and others in an advocacy situation. The novice advocate may not recognize the range of skills needed. That view that must change or the person will never be effective.

6. <u>Recognize the Power of People: Connect with Others, Draw on Relationships.</u> Most problems that impact the care of clients result from either direct or indirect decisions by people. All advocacy involves harnessing the power of people to influence those decisions. The effective advocate recognizes this and works primarily with and through people.

7. <u>Recognize the Importance of Preparation.</u> Preparation is critical to success. Effective advocates know that they typically have to collect information to fully understand an issues, and then take steps to build support and reduce resistance if they are to ensure a positive result.

8. <u>Build Self-Awareness.</u> Successful advocates are aware of their own agendas and feelings. They recognize how they are acting and speaking and how they are likely to be perceived. All of this self-awareness allows them to have more control over their efforts, making it more likely that all these efforts will support the identified goal.

9. <u>Build Connections.</u> Advocacy relies heavily on relationships and so, over time, successful advocates develop relationships with providers, organizations, clients, other advocates, and other stakeholders who can support their efforts.

10. <u>Recognize Your Own Need for Personal Support.</u> Advocacy, like all of Peer Support, is personally challenging work. Peer Advocates are often talking to people who are in distress. Peer Advocates also work on difficult problems, many of which will not be resolved quickly and some of which may not ever be fully resolved. Given the nature of their work, Peer Advocates need the support of others—family, friends, and other work associates. Successful Peer Advocates maintain awareness of how they are feeling and develop the long-term emotional supports they need.

CHAPTER 3

COMMON MISTAKES IN ADVOCACY

In advocacy, as in other areas of life, it's helpful to know what mistakes are most important to avoid. This chapter includes descriptions of some of the most common advocacy errors. You may have seen colleagues make some of these mistakes, and you may even recognize some of the traits below in yourself. By being aware of these pitfalls, you can work toward avoiding them altogether or improving in those areas where you need the most help. Consider some of the following:

1. <u>The Fatalist.</u> This advocate feels that nothing and no one can really change and so gives up too quickly or too easily. The Fatalist may say she is "just being reasonable," but in reality lacks confidence that advocacy can change anything. The Fatalist's actual goal seems to be to avoid failing, and so giving up quickly is a way to protect against disappointment. Unfortunately, this kind of advocate leaves too many successful battles unfought.

2. <u>The Blind Leading the Blind.</u> This advocate doesn't know how to advocate and so stumbles too often to be successful. He

may be well intentioned, but has little experience or training, and unfortunately, doesn't recognize his own lack of skill or experience. Though he is trying to be helpful, without the knowledge of how to be successful, he underestimates the skills needed to be effective.

3. The Flame Thrower. This advocate confuses being angry with being assertive. She feels angry from the start, often before fully understanding the issue at stake. The Flame Thrower often brings personal anger from another situation to the job—a very serious mistake. Often, the goal seems to be to let off as much anger or frustration as possible, which unfortunately does not help in advocacy. While anger can be a tool of the effective advocate, it must be used cautiously and strategically. Poorly used, anger will destroy that specific effort to advocate and will often burn the very bridges needed for future advocacy.

4. The Rabble Rouser. Similar to the Flame Thrower, the Rabble Rouser seems to rely heavily on the strategy of arousing anger—in this case in as many angry stakeholders as possible. Sometimes the reliance on getting many people angrily supporting an issue seems to reflect a sense of enjoyment of loud, boisterous fights. Other times it seems to be one of the few strategies the advocate knows. Regardless of the reason, the Rabble Rouser fails to recognize that he is using a high-risk strategy with many downsides. The cost to the relationships in the organization is high and it will not be seen positively by those he is advocating with. Long-term loss of trust will typically make this a losing strategy if the advocate wants have a role in future issues.

5. The Short-Sighted Advocate. This advocate loses track of the fact that successful advocacy takes place over time—it is persistence that usually results in the greatest change in the

long run. The Short-Sighted Advocate acts as though she must "win" every battle. She often persists after it is clear that she is not going to get the result she wishes—and does so in a way that damages the respect and trust others have for her. She may act as though advocating is a game or battle to be won. However, it is not a battle between "winners" and "losers"—it is an effort to help someone achieve a goal. There is no "winner," only people all trying to find a solution. Black and white thinking like this is often associated with long-term failure. These types of advocates may "win" some positive outcomes, but they often "lose" the long-term trust and collaboration needed to make change over time, and so everyone "loses."

6. The Hired Gun. This advocate appears to lose all objectivity, fully and uncritically supporting whomever he is advocating for at the current moment. Most disagreements have two sides, but the Hired Gun has no interest in the "other side's" perspective. He sees his job as advocating for the client's perspective, regardless of the reality of the situation. This is also a short-term stance that will undermine any trust the other party has in the advocate. More importantly, this stance does not help the client face the reality of the situation or the complexity of the issues that need to be resolved.

7. The Patsy. Like the Hired Gun, the Patsy has lost objectivity, but in this case the advocate has bought into the views and values of the organization and/or people she is supposed to be advocating to. Sometimes this happens when someone has been advocating with the same organization for too long. For example, patient advocates who have worked within a specific healthcare setting for years are at risk for starting to take on the views of the organization and failing to advocate strongly and objectively. The result may be less hard work and fewer

difficult battles, but also fewer gains for the clients.

8. The Long-Distance Advocate. For a range of reasons, some advocates try to do most (or all) of their work by sending emails and letters, but not actually engaging in face-to-face conversation. While a great deal of work can be accomplished via email and letter, there are a number of substantial risks and limitations to heavy reliance on these forms of communication. Effective advocacy usually involves relationship-building and requires a personal dimension to the communication. Email can lack that personal quality, and at times feels decidedly distant and impersonal. The fact that email and letters produce a written record can give the impression that the advocate is purposely creating a legal record, further chilling the nature of the exchange. What's more, negotiating over email is particularly difficult. By meeting in person, each party can see the other's responses in real time, allowing them to connect and build agreement more easily. Taking the time to meet also communicates that the advocate feels the matter is worthy of the time and effort.

9. The Tunnel-Vision Advocate. Every advocacy situation involves two or more parties, all of whom have a number of contingencies related to how they do their work. They have needs they are seeking to meet, as well as other people and organizations that want and need things from them. The Tunnel-Vision Advocate fails to recognize all of the contingencies faced by the people they are advocating to, focusing almost exclusively on the need of the client. This advocate is often seen as unrealistic, impractical, or naive because he fails to see the range of factors that have to be addressed to reach a solution. While he may feel that these issues are not his concern, his failure to recognize the realities faced by others limits the degree to which he can develop positive relationships with those he advocates to.

10. <u>The Crusader.</u> Like the Tunnel-Vision Advocate, the
    Crusader works from a limited perspective. This advocate is
    on a quest to prove that she is right about an issue, but
    unfortunately, she is more interested in being right than in
    accomplishing something of practical benefit for the person
    she is advocating for. The effective advocate never forgets
    who she is working for and seeks to achieve something
    specific that will help in the client's recovery. When the
    advocate's actions seem more focused on proving that the
    advocate is on the "right side" of an issue than on achieving a
    practical outcome for the client, she has again lost track of her
    role.

All of these patterns have something in common. They all are
due in part to the advocate having limited self-awareness -- they
do not see themselves objectively. This is a challenge for all of
us, but advocates in particular can benefit from honest feedback
from those around them who understand what effective
advocacy looks like. To be successful over time, you will need to
cultivate those colleagues and mentors who care about you and
your work enough to give you that feedback. Many people will
have valuable feedback for you, but will not offer it because of
concern that you won't want it or that you'll feel angry or hurt by
honest comments. You will need to go out of your way to find
those who can give you the accurate feedback you need to keep
your work on track, and then reach out to convince them that
you want this feedback. This will be a challenging task, but there
are few more valuable resources to any advocate than a colleague
or mentor who is willing to tell you the truth.

CHAPTER 4

CLARIFYING THE ISSUE—
TALKING WITH THE CLIENT

Advocacy is like any other complex ability: it can be learned, but learning the key skills requires attention and the motivation to pursue opportunities to practice those skills. The following chapters will identify a range of skills that the effective advocate uses in their work. You are likely to see skills that you already have, and others that you need to develop or strengthen. All will require continued experience and reflection on your own performance, if you are going to be an effective advocate.

Most advocacy efforts start with a client or group of clients (we will refer to the person or group you are advocating for as your "client") who approach an advocate with a problem they want help with. The effective advocate recognizes that what the client initially describes may not represent a full picture of the issue, and has the skills needed to clarify what the real problem is, first by talking with the person who is seeking help. While this task may seem simple, it is often more complex for the following reasons:

- Clients may be upset or emotional when talking with the advocate, impacting their ability to speak clearly about their concerns. This situation creates a challenge for the advocate, who has to both find out about the issue and take care of the immediate needs of the client.

- Clients often have not fully thought out what the problem is. They may not be fully aware, or at least not able to state clearly, what change they are seeking.

- Clients are often not particularly objective in thinking about their problem, and may tell their story in a way that explains their perspective but leaves out key information the advocate needs.

- Clients may not be fully honest in telling their story. Rightly or wrongly, they may feel that if they are completely honest, the advocate will not or cannot actually help them.

ELEMENTS OF THE SKILL OF 'TALKING WITH THE CLIENT'

1. Recognize and Respect the Perspective of the Client. Clients typically come to advocates after a problem has become very challenging. Advocates often see clients who are:

- Discouraged

- Afraid of speaking up and afraid of negative results if they are assertive

- Angry

- Confused—they don't fully understand the issue at state

- Lacking insight into the situation, the other party, or themselves—they don't recognize how they feel and how they are perceived by others

- Not being straightforward in what they are saying

2. <u>Maintain a Helpful Stance: Stay Calm, Optimistic, Empathetic, and Reasonable.</u> The effective advocate sets the tone for conversation with clients. Even when clients are upset, discouraged, or unreasonable, the advocate provides a calm, optimistic, and reasonable tone to the conversation. Advocates need to recognize what that tone feels and sounds like, when they are straying from it, and how to recover it quickly when they have lost it.

3. <u>Let the Clients Tell Their Story in Their Own Words.</u> There are several reasons why effective advocates want to hear clients tell their story in their own words. First, it helps the client begin to feel some resolution. Second, the advocate will learn as much from the way a client tells the story, as from the content of the story, adding to the understanding of what needs to be resolved for that client. Finally, the client feels heard, which reduces confusion and interruptions in subsequent conversations.

4. <u>Identify the Key Facts: Who, What, When, How, and Why.</u> Effective advocates recognize the key content in the client's story: Who did what, where, and when. The final outcome of the advocacy effort will typically be determined by these key facts, and so recognizing them quickly allows the advocate to focus the research efforts, often speeding the process toward resolution.

5. <u>Listen Actively—Communicate Back What You Think You Hear.</u> Effective advocates never assume that they understand the client's concern fully. It is always a good strategy to summarize what clients are saying, so that they can see you are listening, and so that they have an opportunity to correct an error in your understanding.

6. <u>Listen with an Advocate's Ear.</u> Effective advocates know what steps they are likely to take to address an issue, and are listening for the clues they need to start to build their plan.

- Whom will they likely advocate to?

- Will they represent anyone besides this client, and if so, who?

- Who will their natural allies be?

- What barriers to resolving the situation can be identified?

- Whom may they have to appeal initial decisions to?

7. <u>Agree to a Follow-up Plan.</u> Follow-up by the advocate is critical. Before the first meeting is over, you should make clear to the client the next steps you will take, which often include the following:

- What else you will do to collect information and why.

- When you will get back to them about how you will be able to help.

- What tasks, if any, are you asking them to do, and why?

- Thanking them for speaking up and reaching out.

- When appropriate, giving some indication about how you think you can help. This gives the client realistic hope regarding the outcome.

- Avoiding overselling what you will accomplish for the client. Often, the initial conversation with a client in distress creates a temptation to promise too much. Resist this temptation.

Special Situation: When the Client Is a Group.
When you are advocating for more than one person, you will want to attend to a few additional concerns:

- How different the perspectives are among the individuals in the group you are advocating for. While differing perspectives are common, if they are too different, you may have trouble finding an acceptable resolution for everyone. You need to know the reality early in the process.

- Efforts to build consensus among clients with diverse agendas may be a worthwhile task. If you can help them build a common goal, your work will be simpler.

- If you cannot build consensus and your clients have different agendas and expectations for a resolution that you support, your plan will likely need to be more complex so that you can achieve those different agendas. You will likely need to be more organized to pursue multiple goals at one time.

- Your clients will need to understand what you expect to achieve. Failing to let all of them know early in the process what you can and cannot do may lead to unrealistic expectations and eventual disappointment.

- Ongoing communication is even more important with a group than it is with a single client. Be clear on how you will regularly update your clients and how you will continue to monitor their interests and input.

Special Situation: When You Are the Client. On occasion, advocates have a personal interest in the issue they are advocating for. Sometimes they are advocating for themselves alone. Before you do so, you may want to consider the following:

- While advocating for yourself may feel easier at first (you don't have to ask for help, you know the situation, you feel you can address the issue), asking the help of another advocate may be better in the long run. A separate advocate will typically find it easier to be objective and to address the problem with a little more distance.

- You may benefit from the support of another person. While self-reliance is often a valuable virtue, it can be particularly challenging to advocate for issues you are personally connected to. In some situations, accepting help can result in better outcomes for everyone.

CHAPTER 5

ASSESSING THE ENVIRONMENT

Many of the concerns that come to the attention of advocates result from a mismatch between the needs of the client and the resources of the clinical environment. Clients may have a specific perspective on the issue that concerns them, but it is often incomplete. As such, advocates commonly need to collect more information from the environment to understand what the full issue is. The issue could involve people (e.g., clinical providers), processes (e.g., the way patients are evaluated), or the physical environment itself (e.g., the location of handicapped access for clients).

ELEMENTS OF 'ASSESSING THE ENVIRONMENT'

1. Identify Sources of Information About the "Environment." Effective advocates identify the sources of information available to them regarding the environment. Given what they know from the client, they often create a list of other people whose perspective can add to their understanding. They can also investigate whether other physical sources of relevant information exist—such as documents that contain policies and procedures or that reflect organizational pressures and

problems—and finally, which physical environments and equipment may be relevant to the issue. By generating a list of information they want to investigate, they keep their efforts focused.

2. <u>Contact Others Who Can Provide Data.</u> It can be tricky at times to collect information from others on a sensitive or controversial topic. In some situations, advocates won't be able to disclose the full reason for contacting someone. In others, advocates won't want to disclose the full reason, as they will be concerned that the other parties will be concerned about possible negative outcomes of talking to the advocate. Effective advocates know that they cannot lie about what they are doing. They also know that if they speak in broad terms about their task ("I am looking for information about XYZ as part of an effort to help a client/resolve a problem/improve a process . . . "), they will find that most people will be willing to be interviewed. If others have questions for the advocate that cannot be answered because the answers would include confidential or sensitive information, the effective advocate will often simply explain this limit.

3. <u>Interview Others Who Have Relevant Data.</u> Effective interviewing is an important skill to develop, and has some common elements:

- <u>Introduction and Rapport Building.</u> An effective interview typically starts with a warm introduction. The interviewer usually reminds the interviewee of the purpose of the interview. She also strives to set her interviewee at ease by acting in a friendly and relaxed manner. In many settings the interviewee will be appropriately concerned or even suspicious about the "real" agenda of the meeting and of the advocate. To help lower this level of distrust, the advocate can provide all of the information she can about the situation and her agenda. By "putting her cards on the table," so to speak, the advocate shows that she wishes to be as open and straightforward as possible. In contrast, being overly secretive and vague, or acting oblivious to the interviewee's concerns may result in increased suspiciousness and likely will lower the chances of an open and frank interview.

- Setting the Agenda. As part of this introduction to the situation, the advocate should clearly state the purpose of the interview: What information is being sought and why? An agenda will help the interviewee know what information to provide and will lessen the likelihood of long, rambling answers that are irrelevant to the issue at hand. By stating the agenda openly, the advocate is telling the interviewee how he or she can help. Interviewees may also provide an agenda from their perspective—something they want to accomplish—whether it's gathering information of their own or discussing some other issue. While the advocate may not be at liberty to address all or part of this proposed action, it is important to see this as an offer to work together to meet each other's agendas.

- Collecting General Information. Many data-gathering efforts seek some information that is fairly general and broad, and some that is quite specific and often relatively sensitive. The effective advocate often starts with the broader and more general information because it is easier for the interviewee to provide and gives the interviewer a chance to build rapport.

- Collecting Specific and/or Sensitive Information. The interviewer should not only order questions so that they are logically related, but also so that they progress from more general to more specific, and from less sensitive to more sensitive. If an interview breaks down when a controversial or private topic is broached, it is better to have most of the interview already completed so that as much information as possible has been gathered. When asking about information that the interviewee may feel is important to keep private for the sake of the organization, it is often useful to anticipate those feelings by acknowledging them but then adding a reason why it is more important still to share the information. However, do not ask about information that you know the interviewee is not privileged to give you. For example, do not ask for private client information that you do not have permission to gather. If you do so, it will simply make the interviewee more concerned about your knowledge and credentials, as you may seem unfamiliar with the basic rules about sharing patient information.

- Closing the Interview. All interviews involve a process of closing the conversation. Often there is some summarizing of what has been discussed, a listing of any follow-up items that either party has agreed to do (information to be gathered and sent), an expression of thanks from the interviewer, and respectful goodbyes. If the interview has been tense or has included some open conflict, it is often helpful to acknowledge it, but then to point out how the interviewee has been helpful and to express appreciation despite what could not be accomplished. As with everything the advocate does, the closing of the interview communicates respect for the other party.

4. Interview Others with an Alternative Perspective. The effective advocate recognizes that there is always a range of

perspectives—more varied than might at first be expected. It is often helpful to gather information about those variations to document the issue.

Interviews with stakeholders with alternative views will typically follow the same general outline described above. Effective interviewers will often find it easier to draw out differences in perspectives by starting with general questions, but then mentioning comments from other interviews to help respondents differentiate their views. For example, statements such as "I understand that there are different views on this practice among staff. For example, some of the people I've talked to state that this is done consistently while others state that it is not being done at all. Tell me about your experience/opinion."

Effectively gathering accurate data about the environment is often a key factor in getting a positive resolution to a challenging problem. The effective advocate approaches this part of the process carefully, with the recognition that these data must be collected carefully, as they may likely be needed to help achieve a final resolution to the problem.

CHAPTER 6

IDENTIFYING POSSIBLE SOLUTIONS

You now have some of the raw material you need to start to think about possible solutions. You hopefully have a clear idea about the client's concern. You probably have their idea of what needs to change, though that may not necessarily be what you think will be a workable or desirable solution. You have the perspective and input from other stakeholders. It is now important that you start to develop a range of possible changes that could address the issue you are seeing.

ELEMENTS OF 'IDENTIFYING POSSIBLE SOLUTIONS'

1. <u>Consider What Is At The Core Of The Client's Experience</u>. The person approached you because of some feeling of dissatisfaction or desire for change. It is not uncommon for clients to focus on a concrete aspect of their experience and fail to recognize that what made them dissatisfied is something else - how they felt the staff person or the organization treated them, whether they felt valued and respected in the overall the experience. Their unhappiness may actually be rooted in prior experiences that they are not

talking about. If you are to come up with a real solution, you want to be sure that you recognize the real problem.

To help you focus in on what is really driving the client's concern, you can ask yourself a few questions.

- What were the specifics of their complaint that seemed to carry the most feeling?

- Does the complaint stand in for something in the background, e.g. feeling disrespected, feeling lack of concern, feeling confused?

- What would need to change in order to resolve that underlying concern? Would changing the specifics of the event resolve their concern or would they have the same feelings about other situations?

2. Consider Which Stakeholders Have A Part Of The Puzzle And What Their Agendas Are.
Lasting solutions will often require changes that have at least some support from the agendas of any stakeholder involved. If you can generate possible solutions in which key stakeholders see something attractive, they are more likely to support the change being implemented, and more likely to sustain it over time. Take some time to consider the following questions:

- Who has a part of the process in which the problem has been identified? (they will likely have a part in the solution).

- What do they care about? What are their desires, needs, goals?

- How do each of these agenda's (desires, needs, goals) relate to a possible solution of the identified problem?

3. Consider Other Problems or Challenges That Are Related to This Problem, Including Problems With Related Causes and Problems With Potentially Similar Solutions.
It is usually worthwhile to review the nagging challenges that you are aware of in this program or organization. Related problems can be sources of important clues to what solutions will work. Consider what active problems you are aware of and look for common clues to underlying issues. Similarly, different problems that may be solved with a similar intervention can also provide you with some ideas that are not only effective, but will be more popular, as they solve more than just one problem.

4. Look for Solutions To Other Problems That Have Been Successfully Implemented Either In Your Program or Another. Other people have often been looking for solutions to problems similar to the one you are focused on. Their ideas and their successfully implemented ideas are a great resource for your efforts. It is increasingly common for lists of "Best Practices" to be circulated within and between organizations in order to serve as a similar resource. "Best Practices" represent innovative efforts that others have successfully implemented to solve a problem or meet a goal. They are often helpful as sources of specific ideas as well as of broader strategies.

5. <u>Consider What Resources May Be Available For A Solution</u>. Some solutions require no actual resources, while others require many. Take some time to consider what resources, if any, might be needed or helpful to resolve this issue. Think in terms of money, staffing (including trainees, volunteers, and other partners), space, supplies, equipment, informational resource, support, etc. Are there any resources that you know will not be available, and so will eliminate certain possible solutions?

6. <u>Think Creatively</u>. Solutions are sometimes simple -- often the client will identify those as part of their complaint. Many times they are not so simple -- the client's solution often reflects their limited experience or perspective. Similarly, other stakeholders will often not see the full picture and so may not be able to identify good solutions. If the solution was simple, it often would have been implemented already. This has come to you because a simple solution has not been found. So you need to step back and try to generate more creative options. You will want to use your brainstorming skills for this step. Remember the basic guidelines for successful brainstorming:

- Withhold evaluation -- any idea is good in brainstorming - try to not evaluate ideas at this point.

- Go for quantity. By trying to generate as many possible solutions as possible, you will more likely to stretch your creativity and to blunt any natural tendency to evaluate.

- Accept wild or unusual solutions. Sometimes the best solutions sound outlandish at first, or include elements that are unusual. Let your thinking include options that may feel like a stretch.

- Look for ways to combine ideas into new variations.

7. Identify Several Realistic Potential Solutions.
If you have been successful in your brainstorming, you will now have a list of possible solutions, some of which will be better than others in terms of their likelihood of success and their likelihood of being implemented. From this broader list, you want to generate a smaller list of more realistic solutions.

While some situations will call for only one solution, most will have a number of potential strategies that can work. You want more than one, as it will be easier for you to negotiate a solution if you have more than one option. It is also more practical to have several strategies, as others will have a part in deciding how to move ahead.

In thinking about how to construct a range of solutions, it can be helpful to look for a range in size -- include small, medium, and large changes. Similarly, think about a range from simple to complex strategies -- include strategies that have a simple change by one stakeholder, and more complex strategies that include multiple steps and/or multiple stakeholders. When considering larger solutions, look for those that ask different stakeholders to participate in the solution. Shared efforts often mean the burden is divided, and that the credit for any success will be shared.

By this point, you will hopefully have a list of strategies that seem likely to resolve the concern. This will give your next efforts focus and direction, and will often be the starting point of discussion among the broader group of stakeholders. This may still change in the coming work, but it gives you a place to start.

CHAPTER 7

BUILDING SUPPORT

You have now identified a change that you think is needed in your organization and collected information about the issue from your client and the environment. In many situations, your next task is to build support for the change you believe needs to occur.

ELEMENTS OF 'BUILDING SUPPORT'

1. <u>Review the Environmental Support for and Resistance to the Change.</u> You will want to take "the lay of the land" at the start of this effort, so that you have a sense of what you are up against. To do so, you'll need to identify:

   • Which stakeholders are supportive or likely to be supportive of the change, and why.

   • Which stakeholders are resistant to or likely to be resistant to the change, and why.

   • Any influential stakeholders who may not have a stance

toward the change but who might be persuadable and influential.

- Any key factors that seem to be decisive for different stakeholders. These could include a wide range of factors including laws, standards, policies, community expectations, and agreements.

2. Do Your Homework: Look for and Check Background Data Relevant to the Change. Effective advocates work hard so that they eventually know as much or more about the rules and policies governing the organization they are working with than the people they are trying to persuade. This takes time and effort, both in learning about these rules and also in learning how to research new situations. If you don't know the rules, you are at a distinct disadvantage in trying to convince providers and administrators to make changes. They can resist your efforts by simply citing the rules or guidelines—they don't even have to be correct, because you don't know enough to challenge them. Because you won't have time to review all the material you might find valuable, it is important that you have collaborators who can help you find the most relevant information. You'll want to consider several common categories of resources:

- Policies, procedures, and guidelines of the specific program/organization you are working to change. These are the written rules that programs are supposed to be following; they often also include statements about what the program is trying to achieve and what values underlie those goals. You will want to pay attention to all of those elements: guidelines, goals, and values. Each could support your effort, even if others do not. If you are working with a program that is part of a larger institution or even a national organization, there may be relevant guidelines at those higher levels that may support your efforts.

- Local, state/provincial, and national laws and regulations. Laws like the American with Disabilities Act (ADA) or Rehabilitation Acts have specific requirements that organizations have to follow. Other national documents, like the President's New Freedom Act, set national or international directions for healthcare and can be used as a reference point for how services should be organized or focused.

- Professional codes and ethical guidelines. In some cases, the professional guidelines for program staff are relevant to your efforts. Each clinical profession has established guidelines and expectations for its members, as well as methods for enforcing those efforts. If providers are acting in ways that are inconsistent with the ethical or professional guidelines set by their profession, there are persuasive arguments to help them change their actions.

- Clinical guidelines. In some settings, guidelines about how to best provide healthcare for certain clinical needs have been published, usually by either researchers or professional organizations. They serve as a guide for how to provide care and can be persuasive tools as models of ideal care. These guidelines are usually updated fairly regularly, so you'll want to ensure you have current guidelines. They are also not typically binding, so in some situations, providers may agree that they are not following the established clinical guidelines for best care, but will not be willing to change their practice.

- <u>Content experts.</u> If you can find professionals who are seen as experts or who serve as consultants on topics relevant to the change you are seeking, it may be valuable to talk with them. They may have useful input on the change you are pursuing and how to achieve it. They may also be able to serve as an authority that will support the need for the change. These "experts" may have national or local credentials, but the key is to find out whether their expertise can help you in your work and/or will persuade others to support the change.

3. <u>Create and Build Support Among Stakeholders.</u> To build support for a change, you will need to meet with those stakeholders who are, or will likely be, supportive, or at least neutral toward the change you seek. These meetings will typically include the following common elements:

- Identifying the problem prompting your effort.

- Identifying the change you are proposing and why. Be specific but concise.

- Providing a rationale for the change. Here you should bring in supporting information you uncovered in your research, mentioning ways in which the change is consistent with goals of the organization, policies and procedures, professional and ethical guidelines, national trends, and clinical guidelines.

- Identifying what you believe is the rationale for those resisting the change.

- Providing a rationale for the change you are seeking and why it trumps the rationale for the resistance. In general, you will want to avoid painting a black and white picture or portraying those against the change in a particularly negative light. Issues are rarely that simple and so such comments tend to backfire, leading to the impression that you have an overly simplistic understanding of the issue.

- Inviting their response. You are evaluating whether they will support your view and why or why not, so ask about their views and what support they are willing to provide. You may need to make further efforts to persuade them, but try to avoid getting into an argument or a discussion that could end up building more resistance than support.

- Asking for specific help if they are neutral or supportive. This could take a range of forms, but you might want to encourage them to speak out about the issue, to let you mention their support to others, or to join efforts to support the change.

4. <u>Reduce Resistance Among Those Stakeholders Who Are Not Supportive.</u> In some situations, reducing resistance is more important than building support. This can be one of the trickier tasks. In some situations, you will want to meet with those who oppose the change you seek. The steps are similar to meeting with those who are neutral or supportive, but with a few key differences.

It is critical that you approach the conversation with a positive, respectful tone. Reducing resistance can be accomplished in part by helping the other party understand why you are pursuing the change, but also by helping they understand that you are a reasonable person and a stakeholder who shares many of the same goals they have for their clients. There is a big difference between disagreeing and being disagreeable. You'll get more resistance when people have concluded you are disagreeable. You will also want to help highlight:

- The ways in which the desired change is related, at least theoretically, to their goals and objectives.

- The ways in which the change will result in positive outcomes for them. There may be direct and/or indirect benefits for them. Think about these benefits beforehand so that you can point them out.

- Those people and groups that are invested in the change, and who may be concerned with resistance to the change. They need to be aware of the downside of aggressively resisting the change.

- Some of the steps you might take if your efforts are stymied. You need to be careful not to sound like you are threatening them, but at times, it is valuable for them to know what future steps you might take that would create unwanted attention to their resistance.

CHAPTER 8

BACKGROUND WORK— NETWORKING

Given the central role that people and relationships play in advocacy, it is important to recognize that effective advocates have strong networks of connections that they have built over time. Networking skills are crucial if you are going to be an advocate in a long-term capacity, either in a single organization or in a region. You will need contacts you can use to (1) keep informed about current issues in your field and the organizations you work with, (2) provide specific information and guidance in dealing with advocacy challenges, and (3) garner support to help influence people and organizations.

Networking comes naturally to some people, but for most of us it takes work. The skills are rarely taught explicitly, but they are very learnable. Here are the key networking skills you'll need.

ELEMENTS OF 'NETWORKING'

1. <u>Identify Who You Will Need to Get to Know.</u> It is tricky to identify who will be most helpful for you to know. It is important to be strategic, as you are unlikely to develop all the

relationships you may need unless you purposely identify people to get to know, and then actively pursue relationships with them. Some general categories include:

Inside Your Organization

- Peers/coworkers in your program/department

- Supervisors in your program and related programs

- Leaders of other key programs and departments

- Leadership of the organization

- Staff responsible for key resources, such as space, funding, construction, human resources/staffing, vehicles/travel resources, etc.

- Staff with informal power—people who are influential but may not have the title that reflects that influence

- Staff who are opinion leaders

- Staff who are planners and new program developers

- Staff who seem to know what is going on

- Secretaries and administrative staff

- Frontline staff

Outside Your Organization

- Peers at similar programs in your community, particularly those active in advocacy

- Leaders of similar programs in your community

- Formal mental health services leaders in your community

- Informal mental health leaders—people who have informal power and are influential but may not have the title that reflects that influence

- Leaders of other influential community organizations, such as religious, political, and social organizations

- Local, state, and federal officials who may have a role with mental health in your area

- Leaders and staff of local and national advocacy groups, such as NAMI, PRA, etc.

2. Introduce Yourself to People You Need to Get to Know. For those of us for whom introducing ourselves to a stranger does not come easily, a few simple suggestions can help:

- Find an intermediary who is willing and able to introduce you.

- Act warm and friendly—even if you don't feel it.

- Be prepared with a brief explanation of who you are and what you do for work.

- Include some comment about something you share, such as shared agendas, interests, problems, or backgrounds.

- Be a good listener—invite them to talk, and be curious about them and their work.

- If appropriate, suggest a follow-up step—a meeting, discussion, phone call, etc.

3. <u>Find Initial Common Ground.</u> Relationships form most easily when the parties share experience or interests. Think about what topics might be shared and try to develop them. Look for common ground in the following areas:

- Work tasks (e.g., "We both have to present at the new employee orientation.")

- Work agendas (e.g., "We both want to see Program X expand.")

- Work experience (e.g., "We both have worked in a hospital setting in the past.")

- Work interests (e.g. "We both love to do community development work.")

- Work problems (e.g., "We both have to deal with this year's terrible budget.")

- Non-work interests (e.g., "We both love soccer.")

- Non-work experiences (e.g., "We both used to live in New York.")

- Non-work problems (e.g., "We both have to deal with the rush-hour traffic problems.")

- Recent news/community events (e.g., "How did you survive the snowstorm?," "What did you think of that election?")

Once you've found some common ground, continue to check in on those shared interests over time, enlarging what you know about the person and letting them know more about you.

4. Connect Over Agendas. In addition to building shared interests, it's also critical to develop an understanding with your connections about agendas related your respective work. This is often the most interesting and energizing part of networking, as you are likely to learn from others and they may learn from you. Use this as an opportunity to:

- Find out about their perspective.

- Share your views.

- Find out what they are planning to do to build on their agenda.

- Share what you are planning to do to build on your agenda.

- Look for and point out areas of agreement.

- Look for and sometimes point out areas of disagreement. This is trickier, in that sometimes explicit disagreement will undermine your connection. When the disagreements are very obvious, it is often worth commenting on them, but in a way that is friendly and respectful, so that they feel that you are colleagues who can respectfully disagree on a specific issue.

- Look for potential areas to pursue both sets of agendas with a shared action. If the agendas are the same, this is not too difficult. But the agendas are different, it may require some creativity—but it is still well worth looking for collaborative efforts. Working together on any type of shared interest is one of the best ways to build lasting connections.

5. <u>Build a History of Cooperation and Collaboration.</u> Networks are built over time—often over the course of years. One of the key elements in strong work relationships is a history of shared tasks and cooperation. Sometimes it will require you to be generous with your time and effort, helping the other person do something that he or she cares about. Sometimes it will require you to ask that person to be the generous one in helping you. Most people enjoy giving to others who appreciate their skill and help. They also like getting help when they need it.

There are others who don't like or are not used to being generous with their time and effort. You may be one of them. These people face a key disadvantage: they either have to get others to help when they are not willing to return the favor, or they have to do everything themselves or pay someone. In none of these options is a network of strong, mutually beneficial relationships developed. When one party asks for a lot but does not give as much, the resulting relationships typically include resentment and resistance. And when one party tries to do everything themselves or pay others to do it, relationships tend not to develop at all.

6. Connecting by Socializing. To develop some parts of your network, you may want to socialize outside of work. This is a great way to further strengthen those relationships and create shared interests and connections, but you should recognize that it also involves a degree of risk. Social relationships outside of work can develop problems that then influence the work. Be thoughtful about when you choose to move to outside socializing.

7. Building Connection through Genuine Respect, Esteem, and Encouragement. In some ways, positive relationships always include the elements of mutual respect, esteem, and encouragement. These happen in a myriad of small and large ways, but effective networkers are very skillful and provide these regularly to others they are connected with. Respect is often noted in how you talk to a person, what you say, and whether you recognize that person's role and accomplishments and the demands he or she faces, given that role. Some people are easy to esteem, while others may require you to look harder for things you like and to focus on those. People typically can read genuine respect and esteem in verbal and nonverbal ways. They can also pick up on fake or forced respect or esteem, so work to find things that you genuinely respect and like.

Finally, everyone needs and likes encouragement. It is important that it be given respectfully and in a way that does not suggest the person is having problems and needs help when he doesn't want to be seen that way. Often, encouragement involves simply communicating that you recognize what a person is facing and that you wish him success in his efforts. It is important to provide the right amount of encouragement—too much and the person will feel uncomfortable, too little and the person will not feel supported. Here are a few simple ways of expressing encouragement:

- Comment briefly on something the person did that you noticed was successful ("That conference you organized went very well!").

- Express a wish for success with an upcoming task or challenge ("I hope that proposal you created gets approval.").

- On occasion, consider noting some skill or quality that the person has and express your appreciation for it ("I've noticed that your program is more organized than almost any other around here—you are very good organizing effective teams.").

CHAPTER 9

BASICS OF PERSUASION

Persuasion is the process of influencing others to do or believe something. It is essential to recognize that persuasion is not manipulation. Manipulation involves controlling others, or causing them do something by working around their choice or will. Efforts to manipulate others typically result in anger and resistance, and often destroy the potential for future advocacy. In contrast, persuasion respects the judgment of the other person, but seeks to influence that judgment toward a desired goal. It is crucial that persuasion skills are used within the context of respectful professional behavior on your part as an advocate.

The effective advocate has a wide variety of tools and strategies to choose from, and thoughtfully selects those strategies most likely to be successful in a given situation. To do so, the advocate considers what the other person cares about and how that individual thinks about his or her work. For some, arguments that focus on the client's recovery will be most persuasive. For others, it may be best to talk about the impact on the organization's budget. Still others might be most open to arguments that link the change to how it will benefit them in their own job.

Regardless of the argument and the audience, there are some common skills and strategies that will help you be more effective when it comes to persuading others.

BASIC ELEMENTS OF 'PERSUASION'

1. Use the 3 *P*s of Success: Prepare, Prepare, and Prepare. Your initial goal should always be to know more about the people and situations relevant to the decision you are trying to influence than the person or group you are trying to persuade. Meticulous preparation gives you the best opportunity for effective persuasion. For example, you dramatically improve your odds of success in a getting a change in a program's guidelines if you know their current guidelines well, and you also know what concerns those guidelines reflect, and what concerns would be raised by the changes you are proposing. Failure to fully prepare communicates a lack of skill and/or caring to the person you are advocating to. Take the time and effort to do your homework before you meet with others.

2. Pick the Right Context to Talk with the Person You Want to Persuade. Context and timing are key. It may not be too difficult to figure out when the target of your advocacy may be most open to talking. However, knowing when that person may be most receptive to talking about the *type* of issue you are raising may be more challenging. For example, asking a manager to make an expensive change right after she just received news that the organization's budget is in bad shape is an example of unfortunate timing. Look for opportunities to talk to when these individuals have reasons to support your proposal.

3. <u>Consider Bringing In Partners With Experience, Expertise, and Resources</u>. You will want to think carefully about whether having others join you will strengthen your effort, or will make the person feel defensive or "ganged up on". Partners can be helpful if they will add important resources to the conversation, including (a) additional voices expressing the need for the change, (b) additional sources of information about the need for the proposed change and (c) additional people willing to offer resources to support the proposed change. If you include others, be sure to prepare them so that both you and they will understand the meeting and what they are likely to be asked to say.

4. <u>Be Organized</u>. Being organized communicates competence, and will gain respect from the person you are meeting with. More importantly, if you are communicating about a problem and/or a proposed solution that has any complexity, you will need to be organized to ensure the other person clearly understands what you are saying. You should be organized in what you say and in any materials you bring with you. Make things easy for the other person to digest.

5. <u>Get Their Attention.</u> You can never persuade somebody who's not interested enough to listen to what you're saying. We all have topics that we are interested in and others that we tend to avoid. Finding the right starting point for the conversation will often be key if you want to have any real opportunity to persuade someone.

6. <u>Build Rapport—Be Likeable.</u> We like people who are similar to us and who like and respect us. This dynamic is both conscious and unconscious. By identifying and

communicating similarities to, and respect for others, you can build a sense of rapport where people feel comfortable with you and more open to your suggestions.

7. Ask Questions—Don't Assume. Be suspicious of your own assumptions about what others think or care about— assumptions are often wrong. Let others tell you what they think or care about: people like to be asked about their views, and this input gives you the most useful information about how to argue for the change you are advocating.

8. Make Comments That Show You Understand Their Perspective. The other person will be assessing how much you understand and incorporate their perspective and concerns in your efforts. You need to make comments that show that you understand how the problem and your proposed solution(s) relate to their perspective, values, and efforts.

9. Make Comments That Show You Have Done Research and Are Knowledgeable About The Issue. It's not enough to prepare for a meeting. You want to show that you have prepared. Mention what you have reviewed or who you have talked to, showing the other person that you've put work into the issue and that you have gained a broader understanding of the problem than they may assume otherwise.

10. Frame Your Goal As Mutual. Win-win solutions to problems are always more likely to be implemented and to succeed over time than solutions in which only some parties gain something significant. If you can frame your proposal as a win-win solution, detailing how both your client and how the person you are trying to persuade (and their organization) will all win, you are much more likely to get a full hearing and to

achieve the change you want. Sometimes this requires more fully understanding the range of agendas that a person and organization have, but it is usually worth looking for those agendas in order to argue how the proposal change will benefit everyone.

11. Communicate Clearly and Succinctly. If you can't explain your concerns and your proposal(s) in a simple way in a fairly brief period of time, you are likely to fail to persuade the other person to change anything. People are often busy and don't have much time to try to understand something you are having trouble communicating. The art of persuasion lies in creating simple, clear messages about the change you want in a way that ties into what they care about.

12. Consider Including A Range of Possible Solutions, Simple to Complex, Low Cost to High Cost, Immediate Impact to Long-Term Impact. When trying to identify ways to resolve a problem, be careful not get locked into one solution. Most problems have multiple possible solutions and most situations have complicating factors that will require that you, and the person you are talking with, entertain multiple solutions. It is also true that people like to make a choice, and will be more likely to respond to your meeting with some action if they have some choice in the matter. Identify a range of possible steps that can be taken. You can frame those steps in a way that favors those you think are most desirable, but by giving multiple solutions you are increasing the likelihood that the other person will engage in the discussion and will take some action.

13. Support Your Proposals With Multiple Arguments. Successful persuasion depends on providing the argument(s) that will convince the specific person you are meeting with.

You often will not know what will be most persuasive for that person. One strategy is to include a range of arguments so that you are likely to include some that will connect with that person. Consider the basic strategies for justifying a change:

A. It is the right thing to do (concern for moral/ethical principal).

B. It is in the client's best interest (concern for the client).

C. It is in your staff's best interest (concern for co-workers/subordinates).

D. The change results in an overall improvement for the most people or the community (concern for the common good).

E. The change is an improvement in professional practice (concern for professional competence).

F. The change is an innovation, and could change the field (concern about new ideas, innovation, and improvement).

G. The change is an innovation and could cause you to influence the broader field of practice (concern about influence and reputation).

H. The change will increase your performance on specific measures of performance (concern about performance, approval of superiors).

I. The change will result in you or your organization getting things that you want, such as money, resources, clients, fame, relative success, etc. (concern about personal/organizational benefit).

J. The change will result in you or your organization avoiding the loss of something that you value, such as loss of money, loss of resources, loss of clients, decline in client satisfaction/loyalty, etc. It could also help you or your organization avoid something negative that is likely to happen, such as client complaints, negative attention from the press or other organizations, etc. (concern about personal/organizational loss).

14. <u>Organize Arguments By Prioritizing What Likely Motivates Them</u>. If you do create multiple arguments for a change, you will typically want to organize them in order from those that you think are mostly likely to persuade the person, to the least likely to persuade. This strategy reflects that fact that you want them paying attention when you present the most influential arguments. If you have done your research, or if you know the person well, you will be able to identify the arguments most likely to persuade, and to select or at least prioritize them in your presentation.

15. <u>Connect Your Argument with Their Beliefs or Commitments.</u> As mentioned earlier, every person and group has priorities (values and concerns) that they are most focused on. If you can shape your arguments around those priorities, you are more likely to get their attention, to tap into more powerful motivations, and to leave them feeling that you understand what their work is like. This task is complex, particularly if you don't know the individual very well. In that case, it's a valuable strategy to talk to others who do know them well in order to find out what beliefs and commitments are likely to connect to your agenda.

16. <u>Inject Feeling In the Discussion of the Problem and Solution</u>. People are most influenced by emotion, though it typically

needs to be presented in a careful and thoughtful way. This has to be done with some subtlety, as over use of emotional language will often result in people feeling that the presenter is either not professional or is trying to be manipulative.

By inserting a few words that communicate feeling, you are more likely to keep their attention, to add intensity to their motivation, and to help them prioritize action. For example, consider the following two descriptions of the same issue.

> "by requiring clients to leave the program after 14 days of treatment, we are putting some at risk for homelessness."

> "by rigidly requiring every client to leave the program after 14 days of treatment, we are inadvertently putting some at risk for losing everything."

The second version includes a few added words that inject feeling and urgency into the description without feeling exaggerated or manipulative.

17. <u>Include Data To Justify Your Perspective</u>. Professional staff are increasingly expected to use data to guide their decisions. This is a positive move, as well-chosen data is more likely to tell us what is really happening in a situation. If you have data available to support your view of the problem or to support your suggested solution, you will want to include it. Be careful to select data that you and the person you are meeting with will see as reliable and relevant. Avoid data that will raise more questions than it answers, or that point to other issues that compete with your proposal.

18. <u>Tap Into Personal Experience -- Theirs and Yours</u>. While the use of data is more likely to tell us about what is actually

happening, there is extensive research showing that people, even highly educated people, are still more influenced by stories of personal experience -- particularly their own experience. If you know that the person you are meeting with has had a personal experience with the problem or your proposed solution, bring that experience back to their mind. The strength of that experience will often increase their interest in the issue.

19. <u>Be Ready With Anecdotes Documenting the Need</u>. If neither you, nor the person you are talking with, has had a personal experience of the problem or the proposed solution, you will want to collect some anecdotes of other people who have. An effective anecdote helps highlight an issue, and gives an example of the subjective experience with either the problem or the solution. You want to be careful, as anecdotes may represent the exception of most people's experience. For example, if a manager knows that a program has high satisfaction among clients, telling an anecdote of a dissatisfied client may not be persuasive.

20. <u>Look For and Refer to Authorities Who Support Your View.</u> We all are more likely to change when we know that many people support a change, and particularly when people we know and respect want the change. Look for authorities who support the change you seek and identify those whose voice would have the most impact on the person you are talking with. Mention that authority's support and, if appropriate, offer to set up a conversation so that you can all talk over the issue.

21. <u>When Possible, Use Visual Images to Build Persuasive Power.</u> What we see is often more influential than what we hear. Recent anti-smoking TV ads use graphic images of the

consequences of smoking and have much greater persuasive power than those that rely on spoken arguments. Take the time to consider whether you can create any visual images as part of your argument—and whether you can do so in a way that feels appropriate and professional. Sometimes, it can be in the form of testimonials, either in person or on film, of consumers who are struggling or have benefited from the proposed change. Sometimes it can be in the form of a chart or table summarizing relevant research findings or other evaluation data supporting the change. If it is possible to do this in a reasonable and clear manner, use this powerful tool to supplement your efforts.

22. <u>Create a Sense of Need, a Sense of Scarcity, or a Sense of Urgency.</u> Most professionals have numerous pressing issues they are working on at any one time. If you can create a sense of urgency around the issue you are advocating for, it helps you compete for their attention and garner the energy that will be needed to get them to follow through. Point out how the change reflects a need in your client, in many other clients, in the organization, among staff, and/or within the field. Point out the negative consequences of leaving the problem unsolved or delaying the resolution, and how those consequences will pile up to create larger problems. Help the person feel the urgency behind the issue by using language that identifies the resulting problems that are left unresolved.

23. <u>Create Peer Pressure.</u> We are all influenced by what we think our peers are doing - we don't want to fall behind our competitors or colleagues. By identifying ways that a problem represents a failure to keep up with the community standard of practice, you can motivate a person to attend to your concern. By identifying how a change you want, is already an

established practice among Peer organizations, you can create powerful pressure to implement the change

24. Frame the Issue As a Story. Good advocacy is often dependent on telling a compelling story. Be thoughtful about how you tell the story of the problem and your proposed solution so that it frames the issue in a way that will motivate others to action. A good story has key characters who face a problem, and who do or will overcome the problem. The story suffers if it is too complex, leaves out important characters or issues, does not have enough tension around the problem, or has no potential resolution. A good story is framed around several key motives of the characters -- they are trying to solve the problem because they care about their clients, or they want to beat their competition, etc. It is often useful to think of different ways to frame your story before selecting the most likely to use. You may also want to have a short "elevator" version of the story, as well as a longer version for use in full discussions.

25. Strategically Use Overstating or Understating. We routinely use language in a way that communicates importance as much as information. It is common to use hyperbole or overstatement to make a point, such as when we say a movie is the "worst/best I've ever seen". Overstatement can be a useful strategy for getting someone's attention and communicating importance. When it is overdone, it can create skepticism and resistance in the other person.

Understatement (describing a problem in more subdued terms) can also be a useful strategy. Understatement of an issue that clearly merits stronger language can also be a useful strategy, often causing the other person to experience the stronger feeling that is understated. It can also help you by expressing your efforts maintain objectivity. When understatement is poorly done, it can actually result in less concern, as the person accepts the understatement as an accurate appraisal.

26. <u>Recognize Common Arguments Against Your Position, and Preemptively Mention Those Arguments Before Explaining the Rationale for Your Position.</u> Some advocates assume it is never a good idea to mention the reasons against making a desired change. The other party often knows the arguments against making the change and is wondering if you know the "other side" of the story. In many cases, if you acknowledge the *reasons against* a change before explaining the *reasons for* making it, it diminishes the perceived power of the reasons against and proves that you see the larger picture and have thought it through.

27. <u>If The Outcome of The Change You Are Proposing Is Uncertain or Will be Delayed, Work With The Effect of "Discounting".</u> If we compare two similar plans to make a change, one that will create benefits immediately and one that creates the same benefits, but in the future, the plan with the more immediate benefits will be more motivating. Similarly, people will be more motivated to make a change that will definitely create a desired change, than one with less certain success. Psychologists use the term "discounting" to describe the reduction in motivation for a change that will produce benefits that are either delayed or that are less than certain. The perceived value of the change is "discounted", like prices for less desirable goods in the store are discounted.

For advocates, the idea of discounting is important because many of the changes you will be pushing for will create benefits that are (a) delayed -- they will accrue over time, and/or (b) uncertain - the probability that they will be successful is less than 100%. The person you are trying to persuade will discount the value of a change to the degree that they think the benefits are delayed or uncertain.

For this reason, you want to address the issue of <u>delay</u> and <u>uncertainty</u> but including information that will give the person an accurate but optimistic estimate of the delays and/or uncertainty. Emphasize any immediate benefits and any certain benefits. Remind them about any successes that others have found to increase their estimate that the change will be successful.

It is important to note that discounting also applies to the costs and negative effects of a new change. If a change will be costly, those costs will tend to be seen as less important if they are delayed. Similarly, if there are possible negative outcomes of a change, they will be less influential in the decision to the degree that they are seen as unlikely. For this reason, you may want to provide data about how negative outcomes are unlikely and costs are delayed.

In summary, be optimistic in how you talk about the impact of the change you want to make, both in terms of the benefits (they are likely and will come soon) and in terms of the risks/costs (they are unlikely and will not come soon). However, be careful that you are not unrealistically optimistic, as grossly inaccurate estimates will result in others losing trust in your estimates.

28. <u>If The Outcome of the Planned Change is Uncertain: Work Around "Loss Avoidance"</u>. Most of the people you are trying to convince, will be calculating what they may gain and what they may lose by making the change. It is important for you

to recognize that in general, people count losses more heavily than they count gains. Simply stated, in most situations people will be more motivated to take steps to avoid a loss than they will be motivated to take steps to gain something of equal value. Psychologists call this "Loss Avoidance", and it is powerful factor in predicting decisions. This is the reason that many people and organizations make decisions that seem conservative. They naturally value what they have more than what they may gain.

If the change you are arguing for involves giving up something that the organization has, or could result in the organization losing something they value, the other person is likely to weigh those loses more heavily than what they may gain. In those cases, you will need to emphasize all of the gains that will be made and the large value of those gains. At the same time, you will want to frame those losses as reasonable, expected, minimal in size, or that they are uncertain or will be delayed.

Many organizations will be concerned about making a change that may result in a failure. Loss Avoidance indicates that changes that result in something they see as failure would be seen as particularly costly. You want to look for ways to help them protect against viewing the change as potentially resulting in a costly failure. For example, by framing a change as a "pilot project" or as "a first step in trying to find a solution", you reduce the symbolic cost of a failure (e.g. we expect many pilots to fail) and helps the person to feel that the change can be reversed if data suggest it should be.

29. Be Ready To Say What You (And Others) Will Contribute.
As your discussion proceeds about a change you are asking for, you may find that it is influential to identify some specific

actions and/or resources that you or others are willing to pledge to contribute to making the change. This is valuable for several reasons. First, it can reduce the costs that the person is considering as they evaluate the proposed change. Secondly, it communicates your motivation, and that of others, to make the change. Finally, it tends to create pressure for the person to take action. When we offer to take action, the other person feels a natural urge to act in a complementary way. The more specific you can be about what you will provide, the more specific the other person will often be about what actions they will take.

30. Communicate Patience and Commitment. Many changes will require extended planning and labor. In most of these situations, you'll want to communicate that you recognize that the change will take extended effort and that you are willing to be part of that effort. This helps the other person to feel that they are not stuck trying to achieve your goal by themselves. It also helps communicate that you understand the size and scope of the effort and will understand if it takes some time to complete.

31. Stay Calm, Focused, and Professional. No personal quality in advocates is as compelling as confident certainty. People who speak from a stance of calm confidence that they are moving in the right direction have a great advantage in trying to persuade those around them.

When you let emotions or other issues limit your focus or confidence, you will usually reduce your impact and look less respectable and professional. This is particularly important when your efforts are not initially successful.

Occasionally, during negotiations, the person you are trying to persuade may not act in a calm, focused, or professional manner. It is important that you not follow the natural urge to respond in a similar way, but continue to maintain your focus if you want to achieve your goal in the end. Taking, and staying on "the high road" will usually result in the better outcome.

32. Use Anger Strategically—and Rarely. Most people are uncomfortable with conflict. If you're willing to escalate a situation to a heightened level of tension and conflict, in some cases others will back down. In other situations, they will become even more resistant. In both situations, it is likely to have a negative impact on their feelings about working with you and what they tell others about you. For this reason, use anger and direct confrontation sparingly, and don't use them in a way that suggests you are simply losing self-control or feel that you have to get your way. Let the anger be tied to the reason that the change is the right thing to do. Understatement is often a good strategy to combine with anger. Keep a clear head and a focused message, even as you express more emotion.

33. Persist Against Resistance. The person who is willing to keep asking for what she wants and who keeps demonstrating the value of the proposed change is ultimately the most persuasive. In some situations, successful advocates simply wear down the resistance of others, who give in in order to make the advocate go away.

CHAPTER 10

PERSUASION II: LESSONS FROM MOTIVATIONAL INTERVIEWING

Motivational Interviewing (MI) is a client-centered counseling approach that seeks to encourage behavior change by helping clients explore and resolve ambivalence about that change (Miller and Rollnick, 2013). MI was developed within a substance-use treatment setting, but is now being used with a range of clinical and non-clinical behaviors. As a clinical intervention, it is not appropriate to be used explicitly as an advocacy tool. However, the approach includes a number of valuable concepts, highlighted in this chapter, that are very relevant to advocacy and particularly to the effort to persuade others.

1. Approach with a Stance of Respect. A basic assumption of MI is that the person you are trying to persuade is an autonomous individual who is responsible for making his or her own decisions. The goal is not to override or undercut that person's responsibility for those decisions. (Those types of efforts communicate disrespect and usually result in no change and broken rapport.) Instead, acknowledging the other

person's autonomy and responsibility and expressing empathy for that responsibility is the proper starting stance for all advocacy.

2. <u>Anticipate Ambivalence.</u> MI assumes that people are ambivalent about most decisions, even if they don't explicitly express that ambivalence. Think about any change you are thinking about making. Typically, you can easily identify pros and cons that you are considering. We may ignore the ambivalence once we've made a decision, but the reality is that ambivalence is common and important in most decisions.

   Failure to fully recognize the elements of our ambivalence is often a recipe for poor decisions or failures to decide. Assume that anyone you are approaching to request a change, will be ambivalent - should be ambivalent to some degree, about that change. The problem is not that they are ambivalent, but that they are not thinking clearly about their ambivalence.

3. <u>Make Ambivalence Explicit.</u> In order to help others make desired changes, it is often helpful to assist them in making their ambivalence about the decision explicit. This includes exploring their reasons for and against *making* the change *and* their reasons for and against *not making* the change. A tool called a "motivational matrix" has been developed as a way of helping clients identify the costs and benefits of changing and not changing. This tool and the concepts behind it can be useful in some advocacy settings.

   Figure 1 provides a blank motivational matrix and two samples of completed motivational matrices, one for changing a decision about a client and one about making a change in a program. In some settings, advocates simply use the logic of the motivational matrix in conversation, helping the person they are trying to persuade to fully examine the costs and benefits of the change. In other settings it may be helpful to actually create a written document with the elements in a motivational matrix. However it is used, the goal is help the person *fully* consider all of the costs and benefits of changing versus not changing.

Figure 1: Examples of Motivational Matrices

Example 1: Blank Motivational Matrix

	Making the Change	No Change
Costs, Lost Opportunities		
Benefits		

Example 2: Completed Motivational Matrix
Target Change: To Extend Treatment for a Residential Client

	Making the Change	No Change
Costs, Lost Opportunities	1. Added expense of extended care. 2. Lost opportunity to serve another client. 3. Making an exception to a rule may result in more requests and complaints about discharge.	1. Higher chance that the client will be unsafe, will relapse. 2. Lowers the program's success rate. 3. Communicates inflexibility and lack of client-centered values. 4. Risk that the client will complain to others; may hurt reputation of the program.
Benefits	1. Client likely to have a better outcome. 2. Shows flexibility and client-centered approach.	1. Easier to stay with regular procedure. 2. Fewer complaints from staff about exceptions to discharge rule.

Example 3: Completed Motivational Matrix
Target Change: To Include Peer Specialists on All Treatment
Teams

	Making the Change	No Change
Costs, Lost Opportunities	1. Will have to hire 4 new Peer Specialists, costing $xxx for salary and benefits. 2. Will need to find office space and supervision for these staff.	1. Lost revenue due to high client drop-out. 2. Continued problems with communication between staff and clients. 3. Will look less progressive than competing programs.
Benefits	1. Will enhance client-centered orientation of all teams. 2. Will increase peer support groups. 3. Will likely decrease drop-out rate. 4. Will likely increase rate of clients transitioning successfully out of treatment.	1. It takes less work to stay the same. 2. Fewer peers on teams will result in fewer voices asking for changes, which may be easier in the short run.

4. <u>Help Them Consider The Full Range of The Benefits of Change and The Costs of Failing to Change</u>.
   The powerful quadrants of the motivational matrix are the benefits of making the change and the costs/lost opportunities of not making the change. You'll want to help those you are advocating to, to think about the full range of

elements in those quadrants. Consider the following categories of benefits for making a change:

- How is the change the "right" thing to do?

- How does the change advance your mission?

- How does the change result in better practice - higher quality?

- How is the change good for your clients?

- How is the change good for your staff/colleagues?

- How is the change best for the community/organization in the long-run?

- How is the change innovative? How does it break new ground for the organization or field?

- How does the change help you keep up with, or ahead of, what your peers are doing?

- How is the change a means of meeting what others expect of you?

- How does the change help your organization/program acquire desirable things?
  1. More funding
  2. More positive attention and praise
  3. More influence
  4. Greater ease and efficiency
  5. Better outcomes
  6. Better relative performance

- How does the change help the person you are meeting with get (personally) desirable things?

- How does the change help your organizations/program avoid negative things?
  1. Loss of funding
  2. Negative attention, criticism, or scrutiny
  3. Loss of influence
  4. More work
  5. Decline in outcomes
  6. Poorer relative performance

- How does the change help the person you are meeting with (personally) avoid negative things?

You will also want to consider how to help the person fully account for the costs and lost opportunities for not making the change. The questions above can guide your efforts to identify the costs and lost opportunities. For example, help the person identify how the failure to change (1) is a lost opportunity to do the "right" thing; (2) is a lost opportunity to improve practice or quality, (3) results in something negative for your clients or staff, etc.

5. Encourage Change Talk. One of the best predictors of whether people will make a change is the amount of time they spend talking about how the change would help them and how not making the change would be negative. If advocates talk in such a way that the other party is encouraged to talk about making the change, it is more likely that it will actually happen. Sometimes when advocates argue too aggressively for a change, the other person naturally tends to respond defensively by talking about the reasons they don't want to

make the change. This is exactly the wrong outcome. Look for ways to encourage the other party to talk about making the change.

6. "Roll with Resistance." This term was coined by the founders of MI to describe a key strategy. The effective advocate should not routinely counter resistance by increasing the arguments for making the change. Instead, the advocate should use those statements of resistance to help the other person further explore the problem. "Rolling with resistance" avoids causing the other person to "dig in" to the stance of resisting the change, and keeps the conversation going about the costs and benefits of the change.

7. Pay Attention to the Importance of the Change. Just because someone agrees that a change should happen does not mean that that person will take action. In most mental health and social service settings, there are many competing concerns. Once someone has agreed that a change should take place, the effective advocate should then inquire about how important the change is to the person. To what degree is it a priority, relative the other competing issues? For example, the advocate may say, "From 1 to 10, where is this change on your priority list?" If the priority is fairly low, the advocate's job now shifts to increasing the perceived priority, using the persuasion skills described in chapter 9.

8. Pay Attention to How Competent and Confident Others Feel About Making the Change. Just because others agree that a change should happen, and that it is important, still does not mean that they will take action. A key issue is the degree to which they are confident that they, or their organization, can successfully make the change. Most people avoid efforts that are likely to fail, and so will not try to make a change if they

don't believe they have the skill or resources to do it successfully. The effective advocate includes this issue in the discussion, asking how confident others are that they or their organization can successfully make the change. For example, the advocate may say, "How confident do you feel that you/your program/your organization can successfully make this change?" If confidence is not high, the conversation shifts to identifying the perceived barriers to success and determining how those barriers can be addressed. This process can lead to useful problem-solving between the advocate and the other party. It can also be an opportunity for the advocate to contribute by helping others find support or resources for surmounting those barriers.

9. <u>Recognize the Signs of Success.</u> Advocates need to recognize the signs that efforts to persuade someone to make a change are moving toward success. These signs include the person: (a) talking openly about the desire to make the change, reasons for making the change, and plans to make the change; (b) expressing that the change is highly important to him or her; and (c) expressing feeling fairly or highly confident that the person can make the change. These are the indicators of successful negotiations, and most efforts toward persuasion should target these intermediate goals.

<u>A Final Comment about MI and Advocacy.</u> MI is a clinical intervention that many staff and administrators in mental health and social service settings are familiar with. If you use MI language or tools too explicitly or too clumsily, those you are trying to persuade may recognize the tools and feel more resistant to your efforts. As an advocate, you should not use MI as an intervention, but borrow those principles that can help increase the effectiveness of your overall efforts.

CHAPTER 11

PERSUASION USING THE LANGUAGE OF MONEY

It is important to recognize that all organizations, regardless of their goals, have to deal with money in order to survive and grow. Managers have to keep their portion of the organization in good financial health, which often takes a significant amount of their time and attention. For this reason, it is often important for advocates to understand the financial issues the organization is facing and to be able to speak about changes in terms of their financial impact. To do this, most advocates have to develop new skills around understanding and working with financial aspects of any issue.

ELEMENTS OF 'SPEAKING THE LANGUAGE OF MONEY'

1. <u>Find Out How Funding Flows into the Organization.</u> Both Peer Specialists and clinical providers often have a limited understanding of the financial side of their healthcare or social service agency, putting them at a distinct disadvantage when they need to argue for changes, particularly a change that will or may cost money. Effective advocates understand the

financial side of the organization, including how funding comes into the organization. For most healthcare or social service organizations, there are a number of possible sources, with many organizations benefiting from several streams of revenue. These common sources include:

- Reimbursable Services. These are services that agency staff provide to clients. Usually a third party like an insurance company or the government pays them for.

- Funding from Contracts and Grants. Some agencies have contracts to provide a certain type of service, and they get those funds over a period of time to provide that service to whomever comes to use it. Sometimes the funds come in the form of grants, which may or may not have fewer restrictions than a contract, but typically are provided over a set period of time with a specific goal in mind.

- Funds from Agency Fundraising. Some organizations raise their own funds from public or private sources, using a wide variety of fund-raising techniques. These funds are usually more flexible but take more work to generate.

- Funds from Competitive Grant Proposals. Some funds are obtained by submitting grant proposals in a competition with other agencies that are also seeking grant funds. The competition is designed to encourage agencies to create the best proposals possible.

2. Find Out About the Current Financial Health of the Organization. To understand how any change will be viewed by managers and staff, you will need to know the financial health of the organization, or a portion of the organization.

To do this, you will want to be able to access the following sources of information:

- Interview staff and managers about their perception of the financial health of the organization. Staff will often know how the current financial state is seen, which is sometimes more important than what the actual financial state is. For example, if the budget is very tight, but the managers are very optimistic about the financial health of the program, it may be easier to get approval for a change that would cost money. Likewise, the budget situation may be very positive, but if managers are very anxious about the financial future, it may be very difficult to get approval for a costly change.

- Review annual reports and other documents that summarize the overall health of the organization or program. While these documents often have language designed to convince the reader that all is well, they usually include specific data about the financial status of the organization: income, expenses, and reserves. They also typically include data about financial trends over time. This kind of information is particularly important as it gives a picture of what is likely in the near future, which is often key to deciding whether to spend resources now.

- Review annual budget plans and end-of-the-year budget summaries. Budgets provide the details of what is likely to be spent in the coming year. They can tell the reader about the priorities of the manager or organization, and what they are willing to put money toward.

3. <u>Evaluate the Financial Impact of the Change the Advocate Is Encouraging.</u> In some situations, advocates will need to be

able to explain the likely financial costs and benefits of the change they are advocating for. This can be trickier than it seems, as some costs and benefits are indirect and can either influence background variables or future costs and benefits.

The table below provides a sample of a simple cost–benefit statement for a proposal to hire a half-time Peer Specialist to do outreach work. You can see that you will want to estimate both what the various costs of a change will be and what the benefits will be. This exercise is actually very helpful, as it makes the advocate think through all the steps that would be required to make a change happen. It also makes the advocate think through all of the benefits of making a change. The benefits (and sometime the costs) are often a mix of items that are either easy or difficult to put a dollar figure to. You'll want to include both types of items, and different stakeholders will care about each. Some will primarily want to see the financial costs and benefits and to make sure the organization/program is not going to lose money, or at least not too much money. Others will put a lot of value on those benefits that are not easily identified by a financial number.

Sampling of Direct Costs/Benefits That Are Relatively Easy to Estimate

- The cost of labor to do something (salary, pay, etc.)

- The cost of specific supplies and equipment

- The cost of services that would be paid by a contract

- Labor costs saved by a new time-saving strategy

- The cost–benefit of future business gained or lost due to a change

Sampling of Indirect Costs–Benefits That Are Relatively Difficult to Estimate

- Improved health of clients

- Improved functioning/quality of life of clients

- Improved quality of care

- Improved morale among staff

- Improved reputation within the community

- Required office space, utilities, etc.

4. Write a Brief Financial-Impact Statement. Advocates may be expected to speak about the cost–benefit of changes they are proposing. This may mean anything from a simple overview of costs and benefits to a very detailed accounting, depending on the situation and audience. Below is a simple accounting of the costs and benefits of a proposal, organized to quickly summarize the most important factors and to point out that the change should result in a gain in funding for the organization. Each situation is different and for those in which the advocate is expected to speak about costs and benefits, each will require a different method of summarizing the financial impact. Whatever you are expected to present, be aware that you want the presentation to communicate your message. Organize the content and format so that that message comes through clearly. Also recognize that your estimates will be scrutinized by others, so try to be as

reasonable as possible. You may want to get help from others with more financial expertise to help you generate your estimates.

Figure 2. Sample Financial Impact Statement for a Proposal to Add a Half-Time Peer Specialist to Do Outreach to New Clients

ITEM	COSTS
Salary (half-time x $35K/Year)	$17,000/year
Benefits (26% of salary)	$4,420/year
Clinical service to support new clients (50 clients @ $250 average cost/year)	$12,500/year
TOTAL COST	*$33,920/year*
	BENEFITS
50 new clients/year @ $1,000 average reimbursement/year	$50,000/year
Serve more clients	
Improved attendance at clinical programs	
Improved service to the community	
Avoidance of problems caused by continuing untreated symptoms in 50 people/year	
TOTAL BENEFIT	*$50,000/year PLUS . . .*
COST–BENEFIT	*+$16,080/year*

5. Understand the Specific Financial Perspective of Your Audience. Good advocates try to understand the perspective of the person they are advocating to, before starting to advocate. If the change they are arguing for involves financial

costs or benefits, it is particularly important that the advocates understand the perspective of that person regarding finances.

Some people are very conservative when it comes to any changes that might carry a risk of losing money. To them, avoiding the possibility of losing resources is more important than stretching to gain something of benefit. For those individuals, the advocate must emphasize the ways that the risk is minimal and manageable. Other people will place a higher value on the benefits that might be gained, worrying less about the risk of cost or loss. To these individuals, the advocate will want to emphasize what can be gained by a change, focusing less on managing the costs.

Similarly, some people are most interested in short-term changes in finances, while others are more interested in the long-term changes. Like costs and benefits, both short-term and long-term changes are important to talk about, but the effective advocate will know whether to pitch a proposed change based on the long-term or short-term outcome.

<u>A Final Note on Talking About Money</u>. In many advocacy situations, you will feel the temptation to overestimate the benefits of a desired change and to underestimate the costs. With respect to finance, this strategy is often a losing one, as managers are often fairly well versed in costs and benefits and will recognize unrealistic estimates. Overly rosy proposals often undermine your credibility. In most situations it will be more persuasive to provide a fairly realistic, or even conservative accounting of the costs and benefits and argue for the change based on these numbers.

CHAPTER 12

PERSUASION USING THE LANGUAGE OF QUALITY

Professionals and organizations are increasingly engaging in efforts to improve their own work. This is a wonderful development that has resulted in many improvements in care. It is also an important effort for you, as an advocate, to be aware of and to connect with. The work you do naturally falls under the category of "quality improvement". If you can help others to see this, you are more likely to get a receptive hearing.

To begin to see how you can integrate with the organization's own efforts to improve, it may be helpful to start with a few key terms often used to talk about efforts to maintain and improve quality.

Quality assurance refers to systematic efforts by members of an organization to ensure that work is done in a way that meets established goals of quality. Most healthcare and social service organizations have some form of organized efforts to monitor and improve the quality of the work they do. The size and scope of these efforts depend on the size and philosophy of the organization.

Quality assurance efforts typically embrace one of several sets of terms and techniques, most of which have been borrowed from the business world. As an advocate, you will be pursuing changes that will improve the quality of the work done by that provider, program, or organization, so it is in your interest to use the language and logic of "quality assurance" active in that setting. In this way, you quickly tap into ideas and terms that are meaningful to your audience, and you will also find it easier to show that your goals are aligned with their goals. Here are some important terms relevant to quality assurance:

Quality management refers to the systematic effort by an organization to manage its work in a way that improves the quality of its products and services. For some larger organizations, this process is run by a department of quality management professionals who use a range of techniques to help improve quality. For smaller organizations, this effort falls to a few specialized staff, or in some cases, all staff may be expected to help carry out the quality improvement efforts.

Customer service refers to any part of the process of providing services to the organization's customers/clients before, during, and after any clinical or business operation. While not all healthcare and social service providers refer to their clients as "customers," there is a growing agreement that keeping a customer service focus in these settings can help improve the quality of the work and the satisfaction of clients and their families. Outreach and enrollment services fall under this rubric, which means that how we let clients know about our services, how we enroll them, and how we educate them about what services are available are all part of good customer service. Similarly, following up with clients after clinical care is provided, measuring and tracking their outcomes, and communicating with them over time are also all part of good customer service. Clients often have concerns about processes that happen before and after they receive care. Advocates who frame these concerns within the context of what is and is not "good customer service" can often increase the willingness of the organization to hear and respond to their concerns.

Clinical guidelines are written documents that include recommendations for how specific clinical interventions are to be provided in order to optimize patient care. These guidelines reflect the results of a systematic review of evidence about effective clinical practice, as well as an assessment of the benefits and risks of alternative care options. Guidelines have been established for a number of different clinical practices, though many practices do not yet have them. Clinical guidelines are generally seen as an agreement by authorities within the community about how certain types of services should be provided. Advocates can use clinical guidelines as a reference for how services should be provided; however, it is important to note that clinical guidelines are not binding, though most organizations want to operate in a way that is consistent with best practices. For this reason, clinical guidelines can be a persuasive tool for advocates. A table in which you can collect some of the more common sources of clinical guidelines for practices in mental health and substance-use treatment settings that are relevant to your work is included in chapter 17.

Patient-centered care reflects a growing perspective on the part of providers and clients that healthcare and social service organizations should offer care that is respectful of and responsive to the individual preferences, needs, and values of the clients, and that that providers should work to ensure that the values of clients and their families guide decisions related to both the services they received and the way the services are provided. A key element of this perspective is that clients are expected to be a central part of any decision-making about services: they are informed about care options, and they are almost always the ultimate deciders about what care they receive. Many of the issues that advocates are asked to help with reflect failures in providing patient-centered care. Advocates can often gain support from providers by using patient-centered care as a reference point and pointing out how the desired change would be more consistent with this philosophy.

Shared decision-making (SDM) is related to patient-centered care and is the process in which clinicians/providers work together with clients to ensure that the clients make the best healthcare and social service decisions. This collaborative effort usually involves open communication about the best available evidence related to any treatment/service decision to be made. Clients are supported to weigh the consequences of options and to arrive at an informed decision about the best course of action. Disagreements between clients and providers often reflect a breakdown of this process or the perception of disrespect within this process. Traditional models of healthcare and social service provision did not view the client as the ultimate decision-maker, and so some providers may fail to recognize SDM as a current expectation. Again, advocates will find that framing appropriate concerns as failures in shared decision-making will often help motivate providers to address the concern being raised.

ISO 9000 refers to a group of quality management efforts that gained wide acceptance in private industry in the 1980s and 1990s. It is one of the earliest and most widely accepted efforts to achieve and maintain quality across organizations.

Total quality management (TQM) is also a system of quality management that was utilized most broadly within government and private industry, though it was also used in healthcare organizations. It was very also active in the 1980s and 1990s, before it was overshadowed by ISO 9000.

The Malcolm Baldrige National Quality Award is awarded each year by a specialized program in the U.S. Department of Commerce to organizations/programs that ensure continuous improvement, demonstrate efficient and effective operations, and provide a way of responding to the needs and agendas of the range of stakeholders, including customers. This is currently a highly sought after and prestigious award. In organizations that value this award and the philosophy behind it, advocates who can point out how an issue is related to Baldrige Award criteria will find a receptive audience.

Six Sigma refers to a set of management techniques designed to continuously improve work processes. It may be most commonly associated with the now-famous efforts of Jack Welch who used it successfully at General Electric in the 1990s. As part of Six Sigma:

- Continuous efforts are made to achieve consistent results in processes central to the organization's core mission.

- Processes are viewed as measureable, and thus can be analyzed, controlled, and improved. Decisions are made based on data and not impressions or guesses.

- The entire organization must be committed in order for quality improvement to be sustained over time. This includes the strong and public commitment of top leadership.

This model provides advocates some additional concepts to use in their efforts. The focus on consistency is very relevant to the work advocates do. Many client concerns are related to inconsistency in the way services are provided, and so advocates who frame those concerns as failures in process consistency may find receptive audiences. Similarly, the focus on measurable results and data-driven decisions provides opportunities for advocates to point out how desired changes would enhance those measurable results.

"Lean" is a term that refers to another group of management techniques, this time with a specific focus on the systematic elimination of waste. Developed within manufacturing, "lean" tools are still finding a place within healthcare and social service management. From a "lean" perspective, waste is most often created through overburden and uneven workloads. A lean perspective seeks to make obvious which activities add value to an organization and to reduce or eliminate everything else. For the advocate, framing problems as wasted efforts may result in greater receptivity by managers and staff in organizations that are using "lean" techniques.

"Improvement cycles" refers to a group of techniques used to address a problem area and to systematically analyze and address that problem area until it is resolved. These techniques have a lot in common but are referred to by different terms. For example, "PDCA" refers to the cyclical process of "plan, do, check, act." A response to a problem is planned, acted upon, its impact checked or studied, and then the results are acted upon. The assumption is that one repetition of this cycle is often not sufficient to achieve full success, and this cycle is repeated until the desired result is achieved. Similar versions have been described (PDSA: plan, do, study, act; DMAIC: define, measure, analyze, improve, control cycle for quality control purposes). In organizations that use improvement cycles, advocates may want to refer to the need for "a PDCA" to address the desired change they are proposing.

ACCREDITING ORGANIZATIONS

Part of the work of quality assurance staff is to ensure that healthcare and social service organizations meet the standards of practice established by the accrediting organizations relevant to the type of work they do. There are a number of these organizations, but some of the most influential and most relevant include the following.

The Joint Commission (JC) is a nonprofit organization that accredits healthcare organizations within the United States. It has greatly influenced how services are provided over the past fifty years. One of the reasons for its influence is that many state governments in the U.S. require JC accreditation for a hospital to be able to receive Medicaid payments.

The Joint Commission maintains an extensive set of standards for healthcare services, including behavioral healthcare services. By inspecting organizations on a regular basis and evaluating the degree to which they meet those standards, the JC either provides or denies a certificate of accreditation. Most commonly, they provide detailed feedback about what standards were met, partly met, and not met.

These standards are wide-ranging, and many of them are relevant to the concerns of advocates and clients. Key areas of interest include efforts to ensure patient safety, the environment in which care is provided, how providers communicate with patients/clients, how restraint and seclusion are used, all aspects of the use of medication, and how treatment decisions and planning are done. The vast majority of issues that clients approach advocates with are related directly or indirectly to some JC standard.

In most healthcare settings, hospital administrators and staff are highly motivated to ensure that their services meet JC standards. Any advocate who can frame a concern within the perspective of JC standards and accreditation will typically find that staff and administrators are interested in hearing about the concern and in addressing it in a way that would support JC accreditation.

The Commission on Accreditation of Rehabilitation Facilities (CARF) is an international nonprofit that accredits rehabilitation facilities, including behavioral health facilities. For some organizations, it is an alternative to JC accreditation, while others seek accreditation from both JC and CARF. CARF has specific standards for mental health and addictions services in the areas of psychosocial rehabilitation, assertive community treatment (ACT), child and youth services, employment and community services, and opioid treatment. CARF tends to have a more explicit recovery-centered orientation and so their standards may be more relevant to some client concerns than those of JC.

The National Commission on Correctional Health Care (NCCHC) is a nonprofit organization that accredits healthcare services in correctional facilities. It was developed in response to evidence that healthcare provided in these facilities was of uneven quality. The NCCHC has separate standards of care for jails, prisons, and juvenile detention and confinement facilities, and includes standards for mental health and substance-use treatment services. Peer and staff advocates working within correctional facilities may find that being conversant in these standards, and framing concerns in light of those standards, may help gain provider and administrator interest.

There are other accrediting agencies, depending on the location of the organization and the type of services it provides.

Advocates will find it very useful to be aware of how their organization is accredited.

ELEMENTS OF 'SPEAKING THE LANGUAGE OF QUALITY ASSURANCE'

With some basic knowledge of quality assurance organizations and processes, Peer and staff advocates are better able to know how to use the language and factors of quality in their work. Advocates may find the following general strategies for using accreditation standards to help their advocacy work:

1. Find Out What Quality Assurance Models and Accreditation Standards Are Active and Meaningful to the Organization You Are Advocating To.

    Find out what bodies accredit the organization and services by asking administrative staff or examining key documents. Become familiar with those accrediting bodies, their goals, and their standards. The standards are often too lengthy to gain a full grasp of, but many organizations have staff that know the standards well and are responsible for helping the organization pursue them. These staff are excellent sources of information about the standards in general, and any standards in particular that may be relevant to a specific issue the advocate is working on.

2. Find Out What the Organization Sees As Areas It Needs to Change to Address Quality and Accreditation Concerns. Virtually every organization has identified some processes that it believes are relatively weak and that it is working to improve. Knowing what those areas are can help advocates frame their efforts in an area of active concern. To do this, become familiar with the results of the last accreditation review(s). Staff should be able to describe the outcome of the

review and, in particular, the areas in which problems were identified. These areas are often seen as a high-priority for change by top management. Advocates who can attach their concerns to those high-priority areas may find administrators and staff particularly open to discussion and collaboration.

3. <u>If Possible, Identify and Communicate the Connections Between the Issues You Are Advocating About and the Quality-Improvement Priorities of the Organization.</u> Often it is fairly easy to identify any connections between those quality-improvement priorities of the organization and the issues you are advocating for, as the issues are closely related. At other times, it takes some thought to identify the connections. By talking with colleagues and quality-assurance staff, you can find ways to link your issue to existing quality concerns and efforts.

Use accreditation language to frame issues when possible. It is often helpful to mention JC or CARF standards that are relevant to issues that you are seeking help with. This raises the prominence of the issue and may improve the motivation for responding favorably.

In addition, look for opportunities to be included in accreditation reviews. As part of accreditation reviews, JC, CARF, and others often seek to gain direct input of clients/patients, Peer Specialists, frontline staff, and anyone serving as an advocate. Being part of the review can give you an opportunity to provide feedback on key issues. It can also help others in your organization recognize that your voice is part of their accreditation.

CHAPTER 13

WRITING SIMPLE PROPOSALS

In some situations, you may be called upon to write a proposal for a change you are arguing for. While many advocates will not have the background to do this and will not be interested in learning how to write proposals, you may be interested and willing to learn this valuable advanced skill. For this reason, a very basic discussion of proposals below, as well as a sample proposal in appendix B.

GENERAL CONSIDERATIONS

Writing is a skill like any other. You can learn it, but it will take effort. The more you do it, the more you will learn. Some people have natural skills that will make it easier to learn, but effort will be required by everyone to learn this.

Writing proposals is a very specific and valuable skill. If you have reasonable writing skills or a willingness to see if you have any skill in proposal writing, you may want to develop this skill. To learn it, you'll want to work with an experienced person who can help you. It typically takes multiple experiences writing proposals to become skilled, and the input from an experienced proposal-writer will help you learn much more quickly.

You will also want to start collecting successful proposals to use as models. By reading those proposals you can typically see why they were successful, and use those lessons to improve your skills.

COMMON ELEMENTS OF A PROPOSAL

The formats of proposals vary widely, depending on who is seeking the proposal and what the proposals are being used for. They also vary in length and complexity, ranging from a simple proposal of 1-2 pages, to a complex proposal of several hundred pages. You'll want to get clear instructions on what is expected of any proposal you are planning to write. These instructions will give you clear direction with respect to the focus of the proposal, the length of the proposal, the organization of the proposal (headings, topics, etc.), and what you can ask for. Common elements in many proposals include the following.

1. The Problem: You are often expected to succinctly summarize what problem or need your proposal is seeking to address. You will need to understand what types of problems can be addressed by a specific proposal, and what are the priorities with respect to the problem. You will want to describe the problem or need in compelling language that will motivate action by anyone reading it.

2. The Background: You are typically expected to provide background information for the proposal. This information often addresses some or all of the following subtopics.

- The background of this specific problem. What causes or factors can you identify? How long has it been active? What are the direct and indirect impacts of the problem? What solutions have been tried?

- The broader context of the problem. What broader issues are related to it? Is the problem present in other settings? Are there community standards or practices that are relevant to the problem or its solution? Is the problem related to any other problems or any other key efforts by the organization?

- Any additional information needed to understand the solutions that you will propose.

3. <u>Relevant Factors</u>: This section is often used to identify any secondary factors that either contribute the problem, or will be supports or barriers to the proposed solutions. Most problems have many indirect factors that contribute to their existence, and it is often useful to name them. Most solutions to problems will have many indirect effects, and must be planned in light of many indirect factors. Again, it is often useful to name those factors that will help your audience understand the problem or your proposed solution(s).

4. <u>Proposed Solution(s)</u>: In this section you will be expected to give a specific proposal for at least one solution to the problem. This description needs to include enough detail so that the readers can see what will actually be done. In some proposals, you'll be asked to include more than one solution, often ranging between relatively expensive to inexpensive options. In some proposals, you'll want to include the option of not changing anything. This is typically used as a reference point for

comparing the costs and benefits of the proposed change vs. the status quo.

5. Cost/Benefit Analysis: In this section you will be expected to give an accounting of the anticipated costs and benefits of the proposed solution or solutions. You will want to include factors that are easy to assign financial costs to, and those that are difficult to assign costs to (see chapter 11).

6. Implementation Plan/Budget: In this section you will be expected to provide a specific plan for how you will implement the proposed solution. This will often include a timeline of steps needed for full implementation, as well as a draft budget for the plan. This will give your audience a sense of what steps will need to be taken and what the likely timing and costs of implementation will look like.

SUCCESSFUL PROPOSALS OFTEN HAVE THE FOLLOWING QUALITIES

1. They follow the guidelines and expectations set by those seeking the proposals.

2. They are clearly written and well-organized, making it easy for readers to easily understand what is being proposed.

3. They are focused on an important problem that is described in a way that motivates the reader to want to take action to solve the problem.

4. The solution proposed is practical. It is do-able given the resources of the organization.

5. The cost-benefit analysis is reasonably complete, with logical and justified estimates.

6. They are specific enough to let the reader know that the proposal is practical and likely to solve the problem.

7. They are written in a way that communicates that the writer is capable of analyzing the problem and carrying out the solution.

CHAPTER 14

ADVOCATING ACROSS GROUPS OF STAKEHOLDERS

Advocates sometimes have to approach and involve different groups of stakeholders, including other consumers, providers, leadership, and members of the community, in order to achieve their goals. Knowing how to move between stakeholder groups can be a key skill in achieving a successful outcome, particularly in challenging situations.

When you are advocating for a consumer of healthcare or social services, in many situations, the most common groups of stakeholders include the following:

Other Consumers. In most situations, there are other people who share the same concern, or at least the same interest, as the client you are trying to serve. Often these people will be consumers of the same services or programs, and they can assist you in a number of key ways. First, if you organize a group, you can not only serve more people at the same time, but also make it easier to get a response from the organization. The organization will find it helpful to know how many people share the concern you are raising. Second, other consumers may have divergent interests that may be adversely affected by your efforts. You want to be aware of whether your efforts are going to cause undesirable effects for other consumers—particularly before you start taking visible steps to make a change. Finally, other consumers are a great source of information for you; they often can provide a rich background to the issue and a broad sense of the best solution.

Other Providers. If you are advocating to a provider, you may find that other providers have similar interests or concerns. Broadening the group of people you advocate to can help spread the effect of your advocacy. In some situations, it can make your job easier, as other providers may be more likely to engage in discussion and to change. In addition, by including peers of the target of your initial efforts, you may be able to bring some peer pressure to bear on that person, which may tip the scales in your favor.

The Provider's Supervisor(s). In most organizations, it is assumed that if an advocate does not obtain a satisfactory response from a staff person, the advocate has the right to appeal to the staff person's supervisor. You will want to know the expectations and norms in your specific organization, but often you will find yourself talking with supervisors in an effort to appeal the initial decision. Supervisors are, of course, different people with somewhat different agendas and values than the provider. For example a provider may not want to alter their typical practice to accommodate the special needs of a client, but their supervisor may be a passionate supporter of patient-centered care, and may support more accommodations. If possible, you want to understand those differences between staff and their supervisors so that you can most effectively gain support for your effort.

The Leadership of the Organization. In some situations, you may want to appeal a specific issue all the way to the leadership of the organization. In other situations, the issue will require that you start your advocacy with the leadership. Again, it will be important to recognize the different values and agendas that the leaders of the organization hold. They often will have a broader picture of the organization, its mission, and its operations. They may also be more sensitive to the need to keep consumers happy—which can help in motivating them to change. They may also be more attentive to financial issues, so be aware of any financial implications of your proposals. Recognize the demands that these individuals often face and plan your efforts accordingly.

Other Advocates in the Organization. Other advocates in the organization can be very helpful allies in some situations. Consider talking with the patient advocate, consumer councils, the "quality assurance" department, and other Peer Specialists. Don't forget the consumers, volunteers, and staff who function informally as advocates. They often have powerful voices that can help you.

Other Related Organizations. Other organizations that are either in the same business, or are partners to the organization you are approaching, may have a part to play in some advocacy efforts. If the concern is a broad one, similar organizations may face the same issue. By broadening your efforts, you may have a bigger impact in more than one organization. It is also possible that similar organizations have already resolved the issue you are concerned about in a desirable way. Drawing them in, or at least referring to what they are doing, may help persuade your organization to change—organizations feel social pressure too.

The Community. In some situations, the local community has an active interest in the outcome of your advocacy. Drawing on community stakeholders (local businesses, residents, advocacy organizations) may be effective in putting pressure on your organization to change. Be aware that this is often a high-stakes strategy, as your organization's leadership will often be unhappy with community stakeholders being invited into dealing with a problem. They may see this as a threat to their control, and if it may result in negative publicity, they may see it as a threat to their job. So you want to recognize that this strategy is rarely appropriate and often risky.

Local, Regional, and National Political Leaders. At times, local, regional, or national governmental issues and interests are involved. Similar to involving the community, involving relevant political leaders is another high-stakes strategy, which will often result in negative feelings by the leadership of the organization you want to change. Knowing whom to contact and when to use this strategy is critical if it is going to be successful.

Professional/Trade Organizations. Again, in rare situations, professional and trade organizations may have interests related to the issue you are advocating for. For example, some of these organizations oversee the practice of certain clinical professions and so may want to ensure that practices meet their standards. Other organizations oversee the work of healthcare and/or social service organizations and also have standards that they want met. Involving these organizations is, again, a high-stakes strategy that should not be considered without a great deal of thought and input from experienced advocates.

Advocating across various groups of stakeholders is a relatively high-level skill that effective advocates develop over time. Some general suggestions for your planning:

1. Think strategically about which groups of stakeholders to engage in any effort. Before reaching out to any group, consider:

- Who has the most interest in the situation?

- Who might have the most leverage on the issue?

- Who seems to be most logically connected to the issue?

- How will they feel about being involved? Would it have a positive or negative impact on their future willingness to help?

- Would involvement of that group generate additional resistance now or in the future, and if so, how much?

2. Consider the possibility of additional stakeholder groups in an effort to "move up the chain of authority." In some organizations, it is expected that patients/clients will appeal decisions they are unhappy about up through the "chain of command". This is often a logical strategy that you, as an advocate, would want to take anyway. If this is the organization's expectation, it is usually in your interest to follow it, unless a special situation arises in which you need a rapid response or you know top management would want to be contacted immediately. In some settings, jumping up over supervisors can be a risky strategy for an advocate—recognize the risks and potential cost to your future work.

3. Consider the possibility of contacting multiple groups in an effort to "move down the chain of authority." In some organizations, and with some issues, it is actually the people at

the lower end of the chain of authority who will have the most influence. For example, in some situations, involving other clients or frontline staff can be a much more effective strategy for change than moving up through hospital staff. Clients, particularly active motivated groups of clients, can have a powerful voice that organizations respond quickly to. Similarly, frontline staff have a special role in all organizations. Engaging a large number of frontline staff can result in an issue being changed or at least reviewed more quickly than appealing to higher authorities.

4. Consider if it will be effective to engage stakeholders outside the organization. Outside stakeholders have a potentially powerful influence over an organization, particularly if the organization wants to maintain the good opinion or support of the outside group. As mentioned earlier, engaging an outside group can be a high-stakes strategy, with significant risks to the advocate and to the issue. Be thoughtful before pursuing this strategy.

5. High-stakes strategies should be used rarely and only after a great deal of consideration. It is important to note that many people new to advocacy move too quickly to high-cost strategies. This often reflects the fact that they don't recognize many of the other options they have. Relatively new advocates should avoid high-stakes strategies unless they have consulted with a number of experienced advocates, most or all of whom support the strategy. High-stakes strategies should be considered only in the following situations:

- After less risky efforts have been tried.

- After careful consideration of the costs and benefits of all available strategies. This should include consultation with key stakeholders who can help you identify and weigh all of the potential positive and negative consequences.

- When the balance of costs and benefits of the specific situation merits taking the high-stakes strategy.

- When the need is so significant and serious as to merit the negative consequences that will likely result from these efforts. Examples include: when the problem is so egregious that contacting an outside authority is clearly merited in order to ensure patient/client safety or the correction of illegal or grossly unethical behavior.

CHAPTER 15

CONSUMER COUNCILS

Consumer councils are a diverse group of organizational structures designed to ensure that consumers/clients have a means of providing feedback about services they have received, with a particular focus on identifying problems in those services, and encouraging ongoing improvement, typically from a client-centered perspective.

Consumer councils can be key influential bodies that enhance the functioning of healthcare and social service organizations by focusing on shared goals related to how services are provided and by creating a venue in which both problems and solutions are made public. On the other hand, consumer councils can also be empty symbols of concern that actually don't accomplish much and thus undermine the confidence of clients and staff that change is possible.

The impact of any consumer council is due in part to the skills of its members. If you have the privilege of serving on a consumer council, you'll want to bring energy, focus, and skill to that role.

Effective Consumer Councils:

- Are made up of a combination of people who work together to improve clinical and social services. Common members include current and former consumers of the service/program, family members of consumers, Peer Specialists, program staff, program leadership, quality assurance staff, and other stakeholders who have an interest in the success of the program.

- Meet on a regular basis in a comfortable space that is suitable for the work they need to do and that communicates respect for the mission of the council.

- Maintain records of their efforts in the form of minutes, and share these minutes with other parts of the organization. These minutes document the efforts to address concerns, and therefore represent a formal and legal record of activity. Formal minutes are a statement to the larger organization and its clientele about the seriousness with which the consumer council takes it role and its work.

- Keep a persistent focus on making real improvements in the organization. There are always temptations to engage in discussion and work unrelated to substantive improvement. It takes a level of focus by the leadership and members of any consumer council to keep the group working actively on real problems.

- Maintain continuous attention to important issues. In other words, good consumer councils follow-up on efforts over time to ensure that a good outcome is reached in a timely manner.

- Are careful to create opportunities at every meeting for members and visitors to raise new issues. Issues can arise within an organization fairly quickly. Unless councils are disciplined, it is easy to become inconsistent in soliciting the latest concerns.

- Achieve solutions to problems, keep track of those accomplishments, and share them routinely with others. Being able to tell others about council accomplishments raises realistic hope that the council can produce real improvements. Describing key accomplishments at the beginning of each meeting and in annual summary reports is a good discipline.

- Regularly invite non-members to council meetings. For councils to be able to influence the larger organization, they need to let others know what they are doing. The best way for consumers and staff to see the council's work is to be invited to attend a meeting, either to provide information about a relevant concern or to provide ideas for needed changes. Invitations to program, service, or organization leadership are valuable for the same reason.

- Take time at least once per year to review how the council is doing its work, what it is successful at, and what challenges need to be addressed to improve its functioning. An annual retreat or review is one strategy to ensure that members and non-members make time to think about how to support and improve the council.

- Pick their battles. No council will work on every issue that arises. There are usually too many issues, or too much variety in the type of issue, for any single council. A seasoned council knows that it must prioritize its efforts if it to be successful on some of the more challenging issues.

- Recognize that success is determined mostly by the willingness of council members to work hard. Significant changes require a lot of effort over time, and a council that takes its role seriously is willing to put in the work required to achieve the successes it seeks.

Common Practices of Effective Consumer Councils:
Consumer councils vary widely in how they operate, and yet councils that are effective over time tend to follow some common practices:

1. Membership
Who serves on a consumer council varies widely, but membership typically reflects two concerns: (a) what groups of people/perspectives should be represented and (b) what individuals have the motivation and skill to get things done. Some common types of members to include:

- Consumers. This is usually the largest group of members. You'll want current and/or past consumers of the services being reviewed. Ideally, these members are aware of the way the program currently functions, are willing to speak openly about issues it has, and are willing to help solve those issues.

- Family Members. Family members of past or present consumers represent a key group of stakeholders whose views are often particularly helpful. Family members experience services from a different perspective, and so can bring fresh ideas for improvement.

- Staff Member Liaisons. It is typically helpful to include staff from the target programs as liaisons for the council. They contribute valuable background information about the problems that have been identified, help with communication between the council and the program, and serve as a symbol of the staff's willingness to listen to consumers in order to improve the program. These members have to be selected carefully to ensure they are comfortable with discussions regarding the need for improvement and willing to help contribute to efforts to address those needs. Defensive or passive staff liaisons can stymie the effectiveness of any consumer council.

- Consumer Advocates. Some consumer councils include members who are not directly aligned with the program, but are consumer advocates. Peer Specialists are often looked to for this role. They can help maintain the flow of information from consumers to the council and sustain the momentum of improvement efforts.

- Other Community Stakeholders. In some situations, it is helpful to include community stakeholders from key community groups or organizations. They may be key partners who will be affected by changes in the program, or they may be groups of community members who are invested in the success of the program.

- Quality Assurance Staff. Because consumer councils are a key tool for continuous improvement, some councils include a member or liaison with the quality assurance department. These individuals can bring expertise in systems improvement and may also help with communication between the organization and the council.

- Consultants and Other Liaisons. Some consumer councils will include consultants and other kinds of liaisons with experience or roles that give them a perspective or information that is particularly important to the council's work. This can be done on a temporary basis to help with a specific issue, or on a longer-term basis. This is an underused strategy that often helps bring the needed expertise and information to the council to allow it to solve particularly challenging issues.

2. Leadership

For any working group of people, good leadership is important. While the group members will typically do most of the work, to be effective a group needs someone who is ultimately responsible for ensuring the group stays on track and that deadlocked issues are resolved.

- Selection. Consumer council chairs are usually current or past consumers who have earned the trust of the rest of the council through prior work on the council. They are usually selected in a systematic manner, such as a council vote. If the chair is appointed by clinical staff or administrators, there will naturally be questions about the independence and authority of the council. These questions are more serious if non-consumers are placed in the role of leadership.

- Role. There are many styles of leadership, and what the council chair does will depend on that individual's style, the needs of the council, and the situation. It is common for the chair to organize the agenda for meetings, and to ensure that housekeeping issues like recruiting new members, saying goodbye to departing members, and maintaining paperwork all get done. More importantly, the chair is often the key person overseeing the functioning of the council and helping it make any changes needed to ensure it is an active and healthy group. Common efforts include resolving conflicts, motivating members, communicating with others outside the organization, creating opportunities to celebrate successes, and creating opportunities to review and improve the council's processes.

- Tenure. The tenure of consumer council leaders varies widely, but should be decided by the council and included in its bylaws. Longer tenure has the advantage of ensuring continuity of leadership over time. This can be particularly helpful if there is rapid turnover among the other members. Shorter tenure has the advantage of ensuring new people with new ideas get chances to provide leadership to the council. This can be helpful if there is little turnover in council membership, and many of the members have the qualifications and interest in serving as part of a rotating leadership.

- Dangers. As with any leadership role, there is the danger that council chairs will use their authority to achieve agendas other than the explicit agenda of promoting the council's work. Sometimes this occurs when leaders want the council to work on an issue of interest to them that is not truly related to promoting consumer issues or client-centered care. Sometimes this occurs more subtly, when leaders seem more interested in using the council for their own personal needs rather than to support the council's work. An example would be a chair who dominates most of the discussion at meetings for some personal need—the need for attention or the need to control. Leaders serve the group they lead, and consumer council chairs must focus consistently on supporting the council in doing their work.

3. Key Documents

Several key documents will support the effectiveness of the council over time.

- Mission Statement. A mission statement is a written document identifying the purpose for the council: what it is supposed to achieve, why it exists. Organizations will naturally shift their focus over time in undesirable ways unless they have tools to remind them of what their focus needs to be. Like a good compass, the mission statement reminds the group and outside stakeholders what direction the council is going in when it is pursuing its true goals.

- Bylaws. Bylaws are a set of rules that a council establishes to govern itself. They provide guidelines for membership, leadership, meetings, and work processes. They also help avoid confusion and resolve conflict.

- Annual Report. An annual report is a key strategy for managing and promoting a healthy consumer council over time. A good annual report will achieve a number of key goals, including:
  a. Identifying important accomplishments of the council
  b. Identifying important needs of the council
  c. Identifying key barriers to the council's success
  d. Creating a sense of continuity for the council's efforts over time
  e. Communicating the council's activity to outside stakeholders

- Meeting Minutes. Minutes document what was accomplished at any specific council meeting, what issues where deferred to the next meeting, and what assignments

were made to council members. Writing minutes may be
seen to be a burden, but minutes are typically associated
with better outcomes and follow-up. Minutes typically
include the following information:

a. Who attended
b. Date of meeting
c. Issues addressed
d. Conclusions
e. Actions to be taken, by whom, and when
f. Plans for future meetings

4. An Effective Consumer Council Meeting

Effective meetings have several common ingredients:

- Established Ground Rules. Whether written or spoken,
  meetings are guided by basic ground rules describing how
  members will and will not interact. Some councils review
  these at the beginning of each meeting to remind
  members. Others review them as needed.

- An Agenda. Most effective councils will start meetings by
  reviewing the agenda for the meeting, including any old
  business that needs to be addressed, and giving members
  an opportunity to identify new business that will be
  discussed during the meeting. The agenda is often in
  written form, and provides guidance for all members about
  how to use the meeting time to complete the work they
  have to do together.

- Respect. A respectful tone is central to any effective work
  group. While many consumer councils represent a variety
  of perspectives, those councils that are effective over time
  are usually characterized by sustained mutual respect,
  including respect by staff liaisons for consumers, and

respect by consumer members for staff and the organization. Effective changes are most likely to happen in an environment of mutual respect.

- Follow-up. Most agenda items that arise at consumer council meetings cannot be resolved in a single meeting. Research and efforts to find solutions will often mean that work stretches across multiple meetings. It is key that any consumer council become very effective at following up on all items raised, until resolution is achieved. This requires that issues are tracked, and responsibilities delegated to specific people and for specific dates of achievement. Patterns of failing to follow-through on items are often a sign of an ineffective council, and lead to low morale and few accomplishments.

CHAPTER 16

POLITICAL ADVOCACY

Advocacy that seeks to influence political leaders, whether locally (town or county), regionally (state or provincial), or nationally, is an important, albeit less common type of advocacy, but one that offers particular advantages. Political leaders are influential stakeholders for healthcare and social service organizations and processes. They are responsible for rules, legislation, and funding regarding some aspects of healthcare and social policy and may have some direct or indirect responsibility for the specific organization that you are seeking a change in. They are also opinion leaders and community authority figures that most organizations do not want to displease. For all these reasons, gaining the support of political leaders can be a highly influential step in any larger advocacy process.

At the same time, political advocacy is also often a high-risk strategy. Unwanted attention from politicians can generate additional resistance to a change. If you are identified as the person who brought political leaders into the process, you may receive unwanted negative attention, and may find that others are hesitant to work with you in the future. Despite these risks, political advocacy is warranted in a number of situations, including those in which:

- The change you are seeking directly involves political entities as key stakeholders.

- The change you are seeking could positively impact larger policy and legislative decisions in desirable directions.

- The potential risks of engaging political leaders in the process have been carefully weighed, and you feel the benefits merit taking these risks.

Political advocacy is a large area of expertise, and a full discussion of this type of advocacy is beyond the scope of this book. However, a few basic principles are worth reviewing:

1. <u>Be Optimistic.</u> Don't underestimate how susceptible to influence political leaders are. Many people feel very detached from political leaders and assume any efforts to influence them will be fruitless. The reality is that most leaders are very attentive to any evidence of their constituents' opinions. Politicians generally like to keep their constituents happy and see this happiness as the key to keeping their job. On many issues, even a single letter or phone call can influence what actions they take. This is due, in part, to the fact that many citizens fail to communicate their views to their political leaders, resulting in greater relative power for the small number of voices politicians do hear.

2. <u>Be Clear About What You Want.</u> Assume that political leaders are busy people with many competing responsibilities. While they want to hear what their constituents want, they also have limited time. Whether you are making a phone call, writing a letter or email, or meeting in person, you want to be ready to state succinctly what you want the representative to do or to know.

3. <u>Be Informed and Credible.</u> It is easier for political leaders to be influenced by constituents who clearly know the background for any request. Specifically, know the background of any problem you are seeking help with. Additionally, know the opposing view of any issue, show that you know it, and explain why you disagree. If you are requesting specific votes on legislation, show that you know the basics of the vote.

4. <u>Be Respectful.</u> You may be asking a politician to do something that that person may not agree with. Do not be uncivil if the politician does not agree to your plan. Engage in discussion if given the opportunity. Do not threaten (e.g., "I'll get all my friends to vote you out of office if you don't support me"), as it is generally not effective and undermines your credibility. Like all advocating, rely on a respectful stance along with the other persuasion skills we've previously covered.

5. <u>Be Personable.</u> While we often hear cynical views that our political leaders are not interested in people's concerns, this is not generally true. Like most people, political leaders respond best when you can explain how an issue has impacted either your personal life of the life of someone else. Including data can help, but often a compelling personal story is the key to gaining their support.

6. <u>Be Connected.</u> Political leaders are not just interested in your views, but who else you represent. Let them know if you are representing a group of people, a formal organization, or common views of a professional group. Advocating as part of a group effort can be particularly influential. Organizations like the National Alliance on Mental Illness (NAMI) organize advocacy events where members and affiliates go together to

state and national government offices and lobby representatives on issues of interest. For those with a particular interest in political advocacy, joining with others through an interest group like NAMI can be a good strategy for building greater skill and influence.

7. Be Engaged. Most constituents never contact their representatives directly, and those who do, often do so rarely. As an advocate, if you develop a relationship with political leaders using some or all of the communication tools available (phone, email, letter, in-person visit), you will have more influence and can actually develop some ongoing interaction with your representative.

CHAPTER 17

PUTTING IT ALL TOGETHER

We've talked about a wide range of advocacy skills at this point. For this book to be useful for your work, you'll need to organize the content and your own thoughts about how to develop your role as an advocate. Here are a few steps that could help:

1. <u>Identify What Type of Advocacy You Want to Do</u>. There are many options available. You need to know what you want to pursue. Spend some time thinking about the following questions: What type of work are you naturally interested in? What options are available to you now? What needs do you see in your environment that successful advocacy could address ? In what ways could you see your interests and the current needs being combined into a real opportunity?

2. <u>Evaluate Where Your Skills Fall</u>. You can make a bigger contribution if you focus your efforts on areas in which you have some skill. Take some time to review the skills listed in book. Chapters 1-9 reflect basic skills that you may need in any work directly with individuals. Chapters 10-12 and 14

reflect more advanced levels of those same advocacy skills. Chapters 13, 15 and 16 reflect skills tied to specialized types of advocacy. You may have a good sense of where your skills lie, but be aware that you may not have had an opportunity to identify existing skills in areas in which you've have had no experience.

3. <u>Specify What Strengths You Have That You Can Capitalize On</u>. People often focus on improving their weaknesses. This is typically a misguided strategy, as you are trying to improve something for which you don't have natural talent. Often the more prudent strategy is to focus on areas in which you have natural strengths, and let those talents work for you. To identify your strengths, consider (1) What you enjoy doing, (2) What do others compliment you on, (3) What do others most often ask you to do. Between these three sources of information, you'll often be able to identify natural talents.

4. <u>What Weaknesses Do You Need To Address</u>? Your weaknesses are still important to consider. If you are clearly poor at a certain skill, and that skill is required for a certain advocacy role, you'll need some method to address the resulting gap. There are typically two strategies. The most common approach is to focus effort and attention on building up the needed skill. This may involve additional training or gaining support from supervisors and peers, as you try to build enough skill so that the weakness does not keep you from being successful. A second and more promising strategy, is to look for a partner or partners who are strong in the area(s) that you are weak. Try to find a collaborative arrangement in which they are doing what you are weak at (and they are good at), while you do what you are strong at. In this way, all elements are done well by those who have a natural talent for it.

5. <u>Develop A Plan For Developing Your Work</u>. If you want to advance your work as an advocate, you will want to be thoughtful about how you go about doing this. Developing an explicit plan will help you be clear about how you will build your advocacy work. Your plan should include several elements. Most important, you'll want to plan how you will acquire additional experience as an advocate. There is no substitute for gaining experience as a means of building skills and influence. You may want to start small in order to start to develop skills. If your experience includes contact with more experienced advocates, your learning will be more rapid, as you get to see others in action. You'll also want to ensure you have regular times of reflection upon your experience. Without reflecting upon your work to find ways to improve it, you are not likely to turn that experience into real skill advancement.

Your plan should at least consider the possibility of finding a mentor. Experienced advocates who are willing to spend quality time with you, working on your development, are key resources to pursue. People are often more willing than you think to serve as a mentor, and so it is worth approaching those who you believe have the skill and experience to mentor you.

Your plan should also include strategies for how to get regular feedback from colleagues and others you respect. If you are to truly build skills you don't currently have, and address the underlying gaps and blind spots that we all bring to our work, you will need colleagues who are willing to look at your work and give you the honest feedback that is required. Many people are not able to be honest in this way, and so you are looking for those who can and will. As with potential mentors, you'll need to approach these individuals directly and ask if they would be willing to give you regular feedback as part of your growth.

Finally, your plan should include ways in which you will expand your learning and skill beyond what your work and the input of others will naturally do. Look for educational offerings, professional conferences, books and articles that can help build your knowledge base. Look for opportunities to try new skills, such as proposal writing, budgeting or working with quality assurance personnel. Expanding your knowledge and experience will often lead to additional opportunities that you are not even aware of currently.

6. <u>Talk To Others About Your Plan</u>. Once you have a plan for developing your work, reach out to others to get their input on your plan. Explain what you are trying to accomplish and ask for their suggestions on how to improve your plan. You are likely to get some helpful feedback, but will also gain some support and allies in accomplishing the plan.

7. <u>Take Action</u>. As is true in all advocacy work, the best plan is worthless if it is not acted upon. Step out and follow your plan. Once you start to move, you'll typically get additional reactions from others and from your environment that will help you see if your plan needs revision. The key is to step out and take action.

A FINAL POINT ON BUILDING SUCCESS AS AN ADVOCATE:

Advocacy is a very special role. You are in the privileged position of telling others how they should change. To truly be successful, you not only need to have a venue in which there are real needs for change, as well as a good knowledge base, good persuasion skills and good networking skills -- you need to genuinely reflect the values you are pushing for. I have had several unfortunate experiences with advocates who are not genuine -- did not act in a way that showed that they believed what they were advocating for. I've have seen advocates argue that clinicians must act more respectfully, but they argued in a way that was disrespectful. I've seen advocates use dishonest arguments to try to convince me that others should be more honest. While they may be right in what they are asking for, it is much more difficult to take them seriously when they don't live out what they expect of others.

As you pursue your work, others will be looking for reasons not to listen to you -- not to have to make the changes that you are pushing them to make. This is natural, as change is difficult and most people feel many competing demands for their attention. If you are not genuine - if you do not live in a way that is consistent with the values behind the changes you are pushing for, you give them an easy reason to discount your input.

Genuineness is a key variable people will be assessing. It is very hard to fake genuineness, particularly over time. You don't want to fake it, and should be concerned if you find yourself trying to create appearances of genuineness. If you commit to be genuine - to truly live out the values you are arguing for - it will be beneficial for you and your work. You will find that it will force you to grow as a person, becoming more of the type of person you want to be, and that this growth will help you become a more effective force for change.

So Mahatma Gandhi's statement "You must be the change you wish to see" is particularly true for advocates, and should be your personal mantra. Think about it regularly. Let it be the core of your advocacy, so that you are always trying to change yourself and others. This will help you empathize with those who you are pushing.

Change is not as easy as it may seem when you are only focusing on what others need to change. When you struggle with making changes in your own behavior, you'll find some of the same barriers that they face in meeting the changes you ask for. Others will then sense that you are aware of the challenges of changing and will see the consistency between what you are asking of them and how you treat others. That sense of integrity, and the respect that it will generate, will be one of the strongest assets you can possibly have as an advocate.

In this way, seeking to become an effective advocate is a journey that requires that you seek to be a virtuous person who works in a way that garners the respect and trust of those around you. The payoff of such a journey is not just a life in which those virtues are present, but a perspective and reputation that will make you an infinitely more effective change agent in the service of others.

CHAPTER 18

YOUR ADVOCACY RESOURCE LIST

This section is designed to help you, your colleagues, and your clients quickly contact people or organizations that may be useful. To be most helpful, take some time to fill in the blank areas in the tables below with contact information for stakeholders that are specific to your position and setting. This may take some initial research, and some effort to keep it up to date, but the resulting resource list will be a very handy tool that you will use many times.

KEY ADVOCACY ORGANIZATIONS

CONTACT	PHONE NUMBER(S)	WEBSITE AND/OR EMAIL
Your state or local mental health advocacy organization contacts		
Boston University Center for Psychiatric Rehabilitation	(617) 353-3549	cpr.bu.edu
Canadian Mental Health Association		cmha.ca
Depression and Bipolar Support Alliance (DBSA)	(800) 826-3632	dbsalliance.org
Mental Health America: National Advocacy Group	(800) 969-6642	liveyourlifewell.org
National Alliance on Mental Illness (NAMI)	(703) 524-7600 NAMI Help Line: (800) 950-6264	nami.org
NAMI—your local chapter *(can be found at nami.org)*		
Judge David L. Bazelon Center for Mental Health Law	(202) 467-5730	bazelon.org
International Association of Peer Specialists (iNAPS): professional association for Peer Specialists		naops.org

CONTACT	PHONE NUMBER(S)	WEBSITE AND/OR EMAIL
National Coalition for Mental Health Recovery: National Advocacy Group	(877) 246-9058	ncmhr.org
Psychosocial Rehabilitation (PSR) Canada/ Réadaptation Psychosociale (RPS) Canada	(866) 655-8548	psrrpscanada.ca
Psychiatric Rehabilitation Association (PRA)	(703) 442-2078	psychrehabassociation.org

MENTAL HEALTH AND SOCIAL SERVICE ACCREDITATION ORGANIZATIONS

CONTACT	PHONE NUMBERS	WEBSITE AND/OR EMAIL
Joint Commission (JC)	(877) 223-6866	jcrinc.com jcrcustomerservice@pbd.com
Commission on Accreditation of Rehabilitation Facilities (CARF)	International: (888) 281-6531 Canada: (888) 281-6531 Europe: 001 (520) 325-1044	International: carf.org Canada: carf.org/Programs/CARF Canada Europe: carf.org/CARFEurope
Accreditation Commission for Health Care, Inc. (ACHC)	(855) 937-2242	achc.org customerservice@achc.org
National Committee for Quality Assurance (NCQA)	(202) 955-3500	ncqa.org
National Commission on Correctional Health Care (NCCHC)	(773) 880-1460	ncchc.org info@ncchc.org

MENTAL HEALTH AND SOCIAL SERVICE PROFESSIONAL ASSOCIATIONS

CONTACT	PHONE NUMBERS	WEBSITE AND/OR EMAIL
American Psychiatric Association	(703) 907-7300	psychiatry.org apa@psych.org
Canadian Psychiatric Association	(800) 267-1555	cpa-apc.org
World Psychiatric Association	+41 22 305 57 37	wpanet.org wpasecretariat@wpanet.org
American Psychological Association	(800) 374-2721	apa.org
Canadian Psychological Association	(613) 237-2144	cpa.ca
National Association of Social Workers	(800) 742-4089	socialworkers.org
Canadian Association of Social Workers	(855) 729-2279	casw-acts.ca
International Federation of Social Workers		ifsw.org global@ifsw.org
American Psychiatric Nurses Association	(855) 863-2762	apna.org
International Association of Psychiatric-Mental Health Nurses	(608) 443-2463	ispn-psych.org

SAMPLE SOURCES OF CLINICAL GUIDELINES

TARGET GROUP	SOURCE/ REFERENCE	LINK
Broad range of guidelines	U.S. Agency for Healthcare Research and Quality	guideline.gov/browse/by -topic.aspx
Broad range of guidelines, including mental health disorders	Clinical Guidelines Office of Dept. of Defense, Dept. of Veterans Affairs	healthquality.va.gov
Broad range of guidelines for mental health and substance-use disorders	American Psychiatric Association	psychiatryonline.org /guidelines
Range of guidelines, adapted for homeless adults and children	National Health Care for the Homeless Council	nhchc.org/resources /clinical/adapted-clinical -guidelines/
Patient-centered care guidelines	Crossing the Quality Chasm: A New Health System for the 21st Century	iom.nationalacademies.org /Reports/2001/Crossing -the-Quality-Chasm-A -New-Health-System-for -the-21st-Century.aspx

CLINICAL GUIDELINES YOU FIND RELEVANT TO YOUR WORK

TARGET GROUP	SOURCE/ REFERENCE	LINK

ADVOCACY RESOURCES FOR ACTIVE-DUTY MILITARY AND VETERANS

CONTACT	PHONE NUMBER(S)	WEBSITE AND/OR EMAIL
Military OneSource	(800) 342-9647	militaryonesource.com
Wounded Warrior Project		woundedwarriorproject.org
Disabled American Veterans	(877) 426-2838	DAV.org
VA Healthcare Eligibility	(877) 222-8387	va.gov/healthbenefits
VA General Benefits Information	(800) 827-1000	benefits.va.gov/benefits
Vet Centers Information	(800) 905-4675 (800) 496-8838	vetcenter.va.gov
Veterans Crisis Hotline	(800) 273-8255	veteranscrisisline.net
Vet2Vet Peer Services for Veterans		vet2vetusa.org
National Resource Directory		nrd.gov
Local/state veterans agency contact (fill in)		

CLINICAL AND EMERGENCY RESOURCES

CONTACT	PHONE NUMBERS	EMAIL
Local police		
Local fire dept.		
Local emergency room(s)		
Suicide prevention hotline		
Child abuse hotline		
Elder abuse hotline		
Rape hotline		
Intimate partner/domestic violence resource		
Pregnancy resource		
Poison control hotline		
Local homelessness/ housing resource		
Local Alcoholics Anonymous contact		

CONTACT	PHONE NUMBERS	EMAIL
Local Narcotics Anonymous contact		
Other peer support group		
In Your Organization		
Your supervisor		
Other supervisors		
Other Peer Specialists		

CONTACT INFORMATION FOR OTHER IMPORTANT CONSUMER ORGANIZATIONS

CONTACT	PHONE NUMBER(S)	EMAIL

APPENDIX A: DEALING WITH CRITICAL SITUATIONS

As a Peer Specialist, you will be in situations where you may have to respond to a range of high-risk challenges. Knowing how to respond effectively is essential for all Peer Specialists, regardless of where you work and what your particular focus might be.

BROAD STRATEGIES

- Learn and follow the local guidelines for emergency responses at your organization. Talk about them with your supervisor so you are clear on all procedures before emergencies happen.

- Practice response procedures so you know them fully. Practice and preparation before an incident will ensure that you know how to respond well when a true emergency arises, and that you can do so while under stress.

- Alert others immediately when you find yourself in an emergency situation. Activate safety alert systems and notify other coworkers. Clinical providers have special training in dealing with clinical emergencies. Get them involved quickly and let them take the lead.

- Try to stay calm. Your ability to think clearly in an emergency will be critical for following through with an effective response.

- "First things first": Attend to immediate safety needs for yourself and those around you before placing all your attention elsewhere.

MAKING A 911 CALL

- Tell the operator what and where the emergency is.

- If someone is injured, tell the operator who is injured and the nature of the injury.

- If there are ongoing dangers in the area that could affect the responders, describe these for the operator.

- Give your name and phone number.

- Do *not* hang up until instructed to do so by the operator.

- After the call, notify your supervisor and/or other key personnel.

- Make sure someone meets the responders and guides them to the appropriate location.

- Do *not* move injured people unless it is absolutely necessary. If medical providers are available, let them decide whether to move anyone who has been hurt or administer other emergency first aid.

- Let the responders do their job once they arrive.

- Document your actions.

- After the event is over, talk with your supervisor and coworkers about how the response went and how it could be better next time.

SPECIFIC SITUATIONS:

A POTENTIALLY SUICIDAL CLIENT

Suicide is one of the top ten causes of death in the United States, and having a mental health or substance-use disorder is one of the most powerful predictors of suicide, suicide attempts, and suicidal thoughts. Peers are very likely to have contact with people who are suicidal, and so will want to seek out training and supervisor guidance on how to deal with this common and critical situation.

If you think someone may be suicidal, contact your supervisor or another available clinician as quickly as possible. Clinical providers often have significant training in assessing and responding to suicidal adults. Get them involved quickly and follow their guidance.

However, it's not always easy to know if a client is suicidal. Someone may need to ask the person for more information before it becomes clear that he or she is at risk. Talk with your supervisor about whether you should notify them immediately or first ask questions of the client directly on your own.

Watch for some of the following common warning signs:

- Talking about suicide.

- Getting the means to commit suicide.

- Being preoccupied with death.

- Withdrawing from social contact; wanting to be left alone.

- Feeling trapped or hopeless.

- Engaging in risky or self-destructive behaviors.

- Increasing substance use.

- Giving away belongings; getting affairs in order for death.

If you are going to speak with the client before seeking out a supervisor or other clinician, ask clear, simple questions:

- "Do you feel like giving up?"

- "Do you think a lot about dying?"

- "Have you been having thoughts about hurting yourself?"

- "Have you thought about how you might hurt yourself?"

- "Do you have the means of hurting yourself available to you?"

If you believe the client is actively suicidal:

- Do not leave the person alone—stay engaged with him or her.

- Get help as quickly as possible. Call a supervisor, 911, or the police, depending on how critical the situation is and who is immediately available to you.

- Keep the person engaged while help is coming.

- Encourage the person to get help.

- Offer to go with the person to get help.

- Be respectful of the person's feelings. Don't be judgmental or patronizing.

A POTENTIALLY HOMICIDAL OR VIOLENT CLIENT

Violence occurs in many work settings, including mental health settings. Training and preparation are critical for recognizing potential risks and preventing violent incidents.

If you think someone has the potential for violence in the near future, contact your supervisor or another available clinician immediately. Again, clinical providers typically have significant training in assessing and responding to potential violence. Get them involved quickly.

It's not always easy to recognize if someone has the potential to be violent in the near future. That's why it is important to take the following common precautions in all settings.

- If you work in a specific area, think about how to make the area safer. For example, make sure you have a way to leave safely if someone becomes threatening. Keep the space relatively uncluttered—eliminate items that someone could use to hurt you or others.

- Have ways to get help quickly, and know how to use them (e.g., panic buttons or alarms).

- Talk with coworkers and supervisors in your area about how you can work together to respond to a potentially violent situation.

- Know how to access security and police officials quickly. Talk with them about working together for safety.

- Request a formal assessment of safety by a licensed professional.

A SITUATION THAT INVOLVES POSSIBLE INTIMATE PARTNER VIOLENCE OR DOMESTIC ABUSE

Intimate partner violence (IPV) refers to physical or sexual violence, threats, or emotional abuse between people who have or have had an intimate relationship. Accurate data about IPV is difficult to collect, but at least 30 percent of women and 10 percent of men will experience IPV in their lifetimes.

Learn and follow the local guidelines for responding to these situations. Talk about them with your supervisor before you uncover actual situations and have to respond.

If you think you are working with someone involved in a violent relationship, or if you think it is likely there is violence, contact your supervisor or another available clinician as quickly as possible. As stated before, clinical providers often have significant training in identifying, assessing, and responding to violence.

It's often not easy to tell if someone is experiencing IPV, and many people are hesitant to talk about it. Watch for some of the most common warning signs that may identify victims of IPV:

- They appear overly afraid of or anxious to please their partner.

- They may talk about their partner's temper or possessive or controlling nature.

- They frequently make excuses for their partner's behavior and negative treatment of them.

- They may have a series of injuries, with vague or suspicious excuses.

- They may frequently miss work or school, again with vague

or suspicious excuses.

- They may be isolated from friends or family. They may rarely see others besides their partner.

The full range of warning signs of IPV, including signs that you are working with someone who may be violent with their partner, is beyond the scope of this pocket resource. Talk with your supervisor about learning more about this topic.

A SITUATION THAT INVOLVES POSSIBLE CHILD ABUSE

Child abuse is common, and can include physical, sexual, or emotional abuse or neglect. Estimates suggest that in the United States, five children die every day as a result of child abuse.

Learn and follow the local guidelines for responding to the discovery of child abuse. Talk about them with your supervisor before you uncover situations and have to respond.

Every state in the U.S. has laws mandating professionals to report evidence of child abuse that they become aware of. Common mandated reporters include physicians, social workers, psychologists, counselors, teachers, and police. Peer Specialists and other people who may not be mandated to report child abuse can report it. Talk with your supervisor and local providers about how to handle situations in which you become aware of possible or likely child abuse. Again, clinical providers often have significant training in assessing and responding to child abuse. Get them involved quickly.

There is a wide range of warning signs of child abuse—a discussion of all of the signs is beyond the scope of this pocket resource. Talk with your supervisor to learn more.

A SITUATION THAT INVOLVES POSSIBLE ELDER ABUSE

Abuse of older adults is also surprisingly common and involves physical, sexual, or emotional abuse, as well as neglect or abandonment, or misuse of the older adult's money or property. Elder abuse can happen in families or in institutions that care for the elderly. Learn and follow the local and regional guidelines for responding to elder abuse. Talk about them with your supervisor before you uncover situations and have to respond.

Similar to child-abuse laws, there are regional laws mandating healthcare professionals to report elder abuse. If you think you are working with someone who might be a victim of elder abuse, contact your supervisor or another available clinician as quickly as possible. Watch for some of the most common warning signs that may identify victims of elder abuse:

- They may seem depressed or confused.

- They are losing weight for no reason.

- They have trouble sleeping.

- They act agitated or violent.

- They have become withdrawn.

- They stop taking part in activities enjoyed in the past.

- They have unexplained bruises, burns, or scars.

- They look messy; they may have unwashed hair or dirty clothes.

- They display signs of trauma (i.e., rocking back and forth).

- They develop bedsores or other preventable conditions.

APPENDIX B: AN EXAMPLE OF A SIMPLE PROPOSAL

THE PROBLEM: Participants in our substance use disorder treatment program would like to have on-site access to specialty 12-step meetings designed to support (a) women, (b) non-religious clients, and (c) clients who are pursuing a harm-reduction model of recovery.

THE BACKGROUND: Participants in our substance use disorder treatment program have limited access to the range of self-help groups that are available in the community. The only meetings available on-site are traditional Alcoholics Anonymous meetings. Over the past year, clients have communicated both on satisfaction surveys, and to the patient advocate, that they would like to have access to specialty 12-step meetings for women (Women for Sobriety - WFS), for non-religious persons (Life Ring Secular Recovery - LRSR), and for people who are seeking a non-abstinence only model of recovery (Moderation Management - MM). This gap in what is offered to participants reduces the motivation of some participants for engaging in 12-step support groups, reducing the efficacy of their treatment, reducing the satisfaction of subgroups of our clients, and reducing our attractiveness to some groups of clients.

RELEVENT FACTORS:
The three partnering organizations (WFS, LRSR, MM) have active groups in the region, and are willing to start up a new weekly meeting on site at no cost to this organization.

Two of our local competitors have already expanded the number and variety of self-help groups available on their campuses.

Participation in our program has declined by 10% in the past 5 years. Participation by women has declined by 20%.

Participation in the programs run by our competitors has not declined over the past 5 years.

PROPOSED SOLUTION(S)

Proposal #1: We could invite these programs (WFS, LSRS, MM) to pilot new weekly groups on our campus for 3 months - each organization piloting one meeting per week in the evening. We will ask them to track attendance. We will track enrollment of women in the substance use program. In 3 months, we will review the resulting data in order to decide whether to make the groups permanent.

Proposal #2: We could collect information from current clients, documenting the number of clients who would attend these groups if they were available. We would then use these data to decide whether to invite these organizations to start groups on campus.

COST/BENEFIT ANALYSIS - Proposal #1

ITEM	COSTS
Space for 3 meetings per week	No additional cost for space
Additional support for security personnel	6 hours per week (2 hours per meeting X 3 meetings) X $75/hour for security coverage = $22,500/year
Labor to track data on attendance at groups	No additional cost -- done by existing staff
TOTAL COST	*$22,500/year*

ITEM	BENEFITS
Likely increase in client satisfaction	
Likely increase in participation in 12-step groups, with associated benefits in clinical outcomes	
Possible increase in new clients seeking treatment from a non-religious perspective, or from a harm-reduction perspective.	We conservatively estimate an increase by 10 clients/year @ $12,000 per client = $120,000
Possible increase in new female clients	We conservatively estimate an increase by 10 clients/year @ $12,000 per client = $120,000
Continuing to be seen as a progressive program that offers clients a high degree of choice	
TOTAL BENEFIT	*$240,000/year PLUS . . .*
COST–BENEFIT	*$240,000 - $22,500= +$217,500/year PLUS improved client satisfaction and increased community reputation*

RECOMMENDATION
We recommend that option #1 be implemented immediately.

IMPLEMENTATION PLAN
1. Dr. Smith will contact the three partnering organizations and arrange for the meetings to start.

2. Dr. Smith will also contact the head of hospital Security to coordinate the beginning of added security for those meetings.

3. Dr. Smith will write a summary report in 3 months, that includes changes in utilization and satisfaction data over the past 3 months, and distribute the report to key stakeholders. The stakeholders will then meet to determine whether the pilot program should continue.

BIBLIOGRAPHY

Anthony, W. A., (2001). *Psychiatric rehabilitation, 2nd edition*. Boston: Boston University Center for Psychiatric Rehabilitation.

Conrad, V. (2012). *Surviving American healthcare: Advocating for yourself or someone you love*. Amarillo, TX: Praeclarus Press, LLC.

Corrigan, P., Mueser, K. T., Bond, G. R., Drake, R. E. & Solomon, P. (2008). *Principles and practice of psychiatric rehabilitation: An empirical approach*. New York: The Guilford Press.

Earp, J. L., French, E. A., & Gilkey, M. B. (2008). *Patient advocacy for health care quality: Strategies for achieving patient-centered care*. Sudbury, MA: Jones and Bartlett Publishers.

Hornbacher, M. (2010). *Sane: Mental illness, addiction, and the 12-steps*. Center City, MN: Hazleden.

Lustig, S. L. (2012). *Advocacy strategies for health and mental health professionals: From patients to policies*. New York: Springer Publishing Co. LLC.

Miller, W. R. & Rollnick, S. (2013). *Motivational interviewing: Helping people change*. New York: The Guilford Press.

Ridley, J. & Newbiggig, K. (2015). *Independent mental health advocacy: The right to be heard*. Philadelphia: Jessica Kingsley Publishers.

Look For The Following Upcoming Titles In This Series:

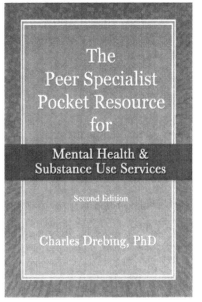

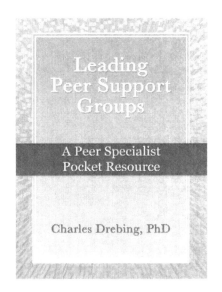

The Peer Specialist Pocket Resource for Mental Health & Substance Use Services, Second Edition

Including Peer Specialists in Health Care Settings is one of the most important developments in the past 30 years. The expanded edition of this pocket resource for Peer Specialists is designed to help you serve effectively as a peer while navigating what is often a complex and confusing clinical setting. Chapters include: Dealing with Critical Situations, Creating and Using Good Recovery Stories, Helping Clients Navigate Healthcare and Social Service Systems, Working Successfully in Healthcare & Social Service Agencies, Good Documentation, Dealing with Legal & Ethical Issues.

Leading Peer Support Groups: A Peer Specialist Pocket Resource

While Peer Specialists are often called upon to develop and lead peer support groups, this is often a challenging task. This pocket resource is designed to help Peer Specialists develop and expand their group facilitation skills to help build and facilitate strong healthy peer support groups. Chapters include: Key Skills for Facilitating a Meeting, Understanding and Maintaining Boundaries, Developing a New Group, Dealing with the Difficult Group Member, Dealing with Difficult Group Situations, Legal and Ethical Issues.

CPSIA information can be obtained
at www.ICGtesting.com
Printed in the USA
LVOW10s0819171117
556676LV00017B/440/P